How I Lost 40 Pounds in 90 Days on the 1200-Calorie Diet

A Simple Plan for Rapid Weight Loss

Cynthia Tucker

Publisher@1200CalorieDiet.Net

How I Lost 40 Pounds in 90 Days on the 1200-Calorie Diet:
A Simple Plan for Rapid Weight Loss
Copyright © 2025 by Clearwater Press
All rights reserved.

1200CalorieDiet.Net
Facebook.com/The1200CalorieDiet

ISBN: 978-0-9890381-3-3
Printed in the United States of America

Table of Contents

Introduction: Three Months and 40+ Pounds!

A re you sick and tired of being overweight? I was, and I decided to do something about it. I had lost weight before but gained it all back....and then some! I was, as the saying goes, all that and a bag of chips … and cookies … and cake—but I digress!

Because I had lost weight once, I knew what to do to accomplish it again—calorie restriction/exercise …. blah blah blah. But there was one difference. This time I wanted results fast. In my first weight loss endeavor, I lost 30 pounds, but it took about a year. This time I wanted, no, I *needed*, results yesterday! You don't need to be all up in my business, but let's just say I was sufficiently motivated. When I found out about the 1200-calorie diet, I decided to give it a try.

You'll want to know who I am and what qualifies me to give advice in this area. Well, I'm not a certified fitness guru, nor do I play one on TV. But can you trust that I know what I'm talking about? Yes, you can. I love to learn, and when a topic tickles my fancy, I go all in to find out all about it. So I've learned all you ever wanted to know about diet, exercise, and weight loss but were afraid to ask.

But here's why you can really trust me—I've actually taken the steps and done the work. This book is not theory, it's not guesswork, and it's not a case of "Do what I say but not what I do." I had a problem, needed a solution, and successfully implemented that solution to obtain the results I desired. I was at 237 pounds when I started the 1200-calorie diet. Three months later, I weighed 195. That's 42 pounds! And quite an accomplishment if I do say so myself. I not only got the results I wanted—I got them quickly. And I'm guessing obtaining quick results is right down your alley.

So I hope my story and the things I learned along the way will help you reach your goals as well. What's even better is that I had several cheat days and weekends, so if you're more dedicated than I am, you can get results even faster. How cool is that? Of course it must be said—your mileage may vary, and you may also lose weight more slowly than I did. Everyone's body is different.

And now for my acknowledgment of the naysayers. Many people are against the 1200 calorie diet and claim we shouldn't eat that little and that it can be harmful. Can it be harmful? Sure. Any diet can. But I promise you'll be fine if you follow the guidelines in this book. You'll be fine as long as you don't suddenly start a vegetarian diet along with starting to eat 1200 calories. Protein will be very important to avoid losing muscle, but we talk all about that and some other things later. I was fine, and you'll be fine too (unless you have medical issues …. then you need to speak with your doctor). So let's carry on.

In this book, you'll learn about how your body interacts with food in the measurement we know as calories. You'll discover your body mass index and basal metabolic rate, all of which can help you maximize your results while following the 1200-calorie diet. You'll identify the real reasons you want to lose weight so that when you have bad days, you'll remember why you started this journey in the first place.

And, of course, you'll learn everything you need to know about the 1200-calorie diet, including how to make it work for you. If you encounter hurdles while on this diet, I've dedicated a whole section to help you resolve the problem so you can get back on track. Through this book, I'll be with you every step of the way, inspiring you to lose those pesky pounds you've wanted to get rid of for so long.

Being overweight is no walk in the park (though it might, and should, result in one!). It affects every area of our lives: our self-esteem, our sex life, and our daily interaction with others. But most importantly, it affects our health. It's a huge problem in the United States and is often taken too lightly. We focus more on how it affects the outward appearance, but the real problem is what takes place on the inside—heart disease, diabetes, high blood pressure, cancer, stroke, sleep apnea, etc. Fortunately, complications due to excess weight are preventable. Many things work together to determine a person's weight, including behavior, environment, genes, height, and metabolism. You can't control your genes or height, but the rest … you're the boss!

The plan outlined in this book is merely one solution to the problem of weight. There are many plans to choose from, and you've probably even tried some of them. If you're anything like me, this isn't your first attempt (though I hope it will be your last).

There are no guarantees in life, but the 1200-calorie diet may be as close to one as you can get. If you decide to try it, you will almost certainly lose weight. There are a few reasons why you might not, and I'll talk about them later.

But for the most part, it will work, and it should work fairly quickly.

Obviously, I'm a woman, so this book is written from a woman's point of view. But you can still benefit if you're a man. The main difference for men will be to raise your calorie intake from 1200 to 1500. You may need to experiment with that number a bit; other than that, there's no significant difference in the steps you need to take.

You've got a life to live. People to see, things to do, and places to go. And when you get there, you want to feel attractive in your own skin. You want that special someone to let out a slow whistle when they see you. You want to be healthy and live as long as you're supposed to. So let's do this!

Chapter 1

Mind Over Matter: The Mindset of Weight Loss

Before we get into the nitty-gritty of the 1200-calorie diet, I want to address something that may be even more important to your health than counting calories.

When most of us decide to lose weight, we're hyper-focused on the way we look. I'm guilty of it too! Hollywood, whether intentionally or not, drills into our heads that we don't have worth unless we're beautiful and sexy according to their standards. So it's essential to reframe your mindset toward losing weight. Maybe you've tried to slim down before and already feel burned out. If so, then this message is especially important for you to hear.

Maybe you're one of those people who uses "tough love" to motivate yourself. If that works for you, I'm not going to tell you you're wrong! However, I do think that kind of motivation can be balanced out with a little more self-kindness. And let me tell you something that may help you see the value in self-care. When you criticize yourself, your body releases the stress hormone cortisol. This hormone increases the buildup of fat around your abdomen, which is the exact opposite of what you're aiming for. Since your body's biology predisposes you to retain fat when you're stressed, it's important that you work to combat stress whenever possible. And being kinder to yourself is an excellent way to do this.

You want to set yourself up for success, not failure, and that's true for the 1200-calorie diet as well as every other part of your life. Ultimately, all battles start in the mind. And you can certainly win this one. I'm going to show you how.

Why Am I Overweight?

Most people gain weight as a result of consuming excess calories and living a lifestyle that includes very little physical activity. However, you may not know about other factors that can contribute to weight gain. It's important that you understand why you gained weight in the first place. Arming yourself with this knowledge will help you address the exact problems that stand in the way of your weight loss.

Emotional distress can often lead to over-eating. Following a death in the family, a divorce, or any other stressful life event, it is not uncommon for people to try to cope with pain by eating more than usual. If your weight gain began around a bad time in your life, it's important to be aware of that. Maybe you need to address emotional or spiritual problems before you can finally conquer those cravings.

Underlying health issues may also contribute to weight gain. For instance, hypothyroidism is a health concern in which your thyroid gland fails to do its normal job of regulating metabolism. When your metabolism slows down due to an underactive thyroid, you will begin to gain weight. If you have diabetes, weight gain can also be a side effect of taking insulin. In addition, a diabetic person may try to prevent low blood sugar by eating more than they need to. The list of problems that may lead a person to gain weight is quite long. Complications such as Cushing's syndrome, fluid retention, stress, fatigue, and even steroid treatment can cause you to gain weight. If you have any of these conditions, try to be as patient as possible with yourself. And definitely consult your doctor before you begin the 1200-calorie diet. It's hard enough to lose weight without health issues that slow down the process even further, so give yourself a break!

As if that wasn't enough, consider how many unhealthy foods are readily available to us. Cheeseburgers, fried foods, candy bars, and pastries can be pretty hard to resist. However, it's important to remember that these foods are created to be addictive. Yes! Manufacturers create these foods to get you hooked! And if you're hooked, you'll eat more of what tastes good. Isn't that messed up? If you eat too much sugar every day, you're going to crave it as if you were a smoker and sugar was the cigarette. So don't beat yourself up if you find it extremely hard to avoid eating fatty, sugary foods. In fact, this diet isn't about giving up certain foods—just about limiting them.

Choosing to Eat Mindfully

Ernest Hemingway once gave the following suggestion: "Try to learn to breathe deeply, really to taste your food when you eat, and when you sleep really to sleep." Though this advice was given to writers so that they learn to pay attention to their surroundings, this is actually great life advice in general.

What Hemingway describes is mindfulness, which is simply the mental state of being completely aware of the present moment. So when you eat, take the time to sit down and really focus on your food. If this sounds obvious, you may be surprised that it's much less common than you may think.

How many of you eat dinner while you watch your favorite TV show? When you snack, are you surprised to find that you've eaten the whole bag of chips because you simply weren't paying attention? I think we've all been guilty of these things at one time or another; it's totally normal, especially for those of us with fast-paced and hectic lives. But when you hardly notice that you've eaten, what's to stop you from feeling hungry again? Studies show that if you eat while you're distracted, you're much more likely to consume more food than if you were actually paying attention. Additionally, it can take your brain up to 20 minutes to realize that you are full.

However, you can approach food in a way that will keep you feeling fuller for longer and increase the enjoyment you get from eating. Make sure your mealtime is wholly devoted to appreciating your food. You can start by turning off the TV. Maybe take the time to try out a new recipe or cook a favorite meal. Pay attention to how the ingredients blend as you mix them. As you fix your plate, notice how beautiful and colorful the food is. Smell the different flavors mingling in the air. Sit down at a table with a glass of water and take a moment to bow your head in thanks and be grateful for your food. Appreciate how lucky you are to be warm and well-fed. Eat slowly. As you chew each bite, really notice the flavors of the food and the sensation of eating. When you start to feel full, stop eating.

When you eat mindfully, you may be surprised to find that you become fuller faster. This is because the act of appreciating your food allows you to pay attention to other parts of your body. Thus, you're more likely to notice when your stomach says that it's time to stop.

If you practice mindful eating long enough, you may even begin to be able to distinguish emotional cravings from true hunger. Emotional eating is when you consume food in response to some emotional experience. I'm sure you're familiar with the common scene on TV where two women commiserate over a tub of ice cream after a bad break-up. As cliché as this might be, it is accurate in its representation—we do use food to cope with emotional distress. I know a little (okay, a lot) about this. I don't grab a tub of ice cream, but I treat myself in other ways. I may take myself out to a restaurant and order the most fattening, calorie-filled dish. Or I might go to Wendy's or Popeyes for a juicy burger or four-piece mild meal—even though I've got lots of food in the fridge.

And this applies to positive emotions as well; rewarding yourself with food and over-eating to celebrate are also examples of emotional eating. We all eat emotionally sometimes, but it becomes a problem if this is your primary response. At the end of the day, this will only make you feel better temporarily. And it will cause you to feel powerless over your food. Mindful eating will help you overcome the impulse to eat based on your emotional cycles.

The 1200-calorie diet WILL help you lose weight, but how will you keep the weight off once you stop restricting your calorie count? I'm going to give you advice later on how to maintain your weight, but if you haven't addressed the root causes of your tendency to over-eat, you're likely to fall right back into old habits. Therefore, you owe it to yourself to develop a new attitude toward eating that will ensure your relationship with food improves. This will help you actually keep the weight off once you lose it.

I am prone to discouragement and depression, so I need to always be doing things that keep my stress levels low and my contentment level high. For me, that's listening to Christian music and R&B oldies, watching old TV shows, playing piano (badly), reading the Bible, and even exercising. Whatever your "thing" is, do it consistently. Don't wait until you're in the middle of a crisis to do something you love because, often, you won't feel like doing it. Keep your tank full so that you'll have the strength to combat those pesky cravings when they come.

So Why Are You Doing This?

I know what you're thinking. *Duh, Lady! I want to lose weight; isn't that why you wrote this book*? Ok, yes, I know you're doing this to lose weight, but you need a more specific goal because you aren't going to stay on this diet for the rest of your life. More than the WHAT (lose weight), you need a WHY! So it's time to do some soul-searching and identify your personal reasons for wanting to lose weight.

Now of course, everyone can come up with at least one less-than-admirable reason for wanting to lose weight. Maybe you want to get a revenge body to make an ex jealous, or you have something to prove to your mother, who is always commenting on your weight. But we've all got great reasons for wanting to lose weight as well. Do you want to be healthier, look better, keep up with your kids when they're playing, or look good for your partner?

Once you've gotten to the truth of why you want to start the 1200-calorie diet, you'll feel better knowing exactly why you're committing to all of this hard work. And knowing your **Why** will help you immensely whenever you come close to throwing in the towel. After all, I know how hard it is to keep yourself motivated sometimes. Maybe you had a crappy day at work and don't think you have the energy to resist snacking in front of the TV all night. We've all been there.

When you reflect on your **Why**, you begin to ask the right questions. Is that cupcake worth derailing your progress? Is emotional eating worth not being able to keep up with your kids on the playground? Remember why you started this journey in the first place, and make every decision with that in mind. This will give you a fighting chance to stay motivated when you're tempted to fall off the wagon.

Motivation

In a perfect world, we would all be motivated to do the things we need to do. Unfortunately, we need motivation to get motivated! We all know how hard it is to motivate yourself to stick to a diet. What if I told you that, with enough persistence and dedication, you could set yourself up for success?

There are two kinds of motivation: intrinsic and extrinsic. Extrinsic motivation ("ext" like external) comes from something outside of us. When we are seeking to reach a goal, such as winning a trophy or avoiding an unpleasant punishment, we are *extrinsically* motivated. In contrast, intrinsic motivation ("in" like inside) comes from within. We are *intrinsically* motivated to do things just because we enjoy them. For example, if you have a favorite hobby like painting or playing the guitar, you probably do it because you enjoy it.

It's important to understand these two kinds of motivation because they affect your behavior in different ways. Most of our motivation to lose weight is probably extrinsic. We want to avoid looking chubby, and we're looking forward to the reward of seeing a smaller number on the scale. There's nothing wrong with that! Extrinsic motivation can certainly help you reach your goals. However, this kind of motivation is most effective when combined with intrinsic motivation. In terms of your fitness journey, you would experience intrinsic motivation when you start making healthy choices mainly because it makes you *feel* better. Maybe you stop being so concerned with where you're headed (weight loss) and start focusing on how good it feels to treat your body well on the way to your destination.

For example, maybe you go to the gym three times a week for a month. At first, you're extrinsically motivated to lose weight and increase muscle tone. Then at the beginning of the second month, you notice that you are actually excited about going to the gym. This is how intrinsic motivation can (and often does) sneak up on you once you've formed a habit. And this is exactly what happened to me. Out of nowhere, I developed a taste for drinking water and looked forward to my gym/exercise sessions. Imagine that!

Maybe you're far from being intrinsically motivated, and that's completely okay. But always be on the look-out for moments when you could take a breath, pay attention to your surroundings, and choose to enjoy the journey. Not only will this shift in perspective increase your life satisfaction, but it will also make losing weight less difficult. After all, if you enjoy an activity, it's much easier to return to it again and again.

Ensure Success Through Compassion

Your weight loss journey demands compassion. If you're not kind to yourself, it will be very difficult to find the motivation to stick to the 1200-calorie diet. Maybe you will get through a couple of weeks but then you notice the scale hasn't moved and you binge eat for the next week.

Let me put it another way. One day, you're going about your merry way, and then BAM! You catch a glimpse of yourself in a store window or a mirror. Right then and there, you decide it's time to lose weight. But you wonder, *Will it work this time*? Instantly, your mind fills with doubt and shame. You feel angry at yourself for letting it get this far. You want to curl up into a ball and eat Cheetos while watching mindless TV.

But trying to motivate yourself by shaming yourself does not set you up for success. Again, practicing self-kindness will help you cope with problems from a place of self-worth and confidence. But this doesn't mean you shouldn't exercise self-control. Sometimes, the best way to be kind to yourself is to set boundaries on your behavior. Fortunately for our purpose, your main boundary will be calorie restriction …. Perhaps not easy, but really simple as to the instructions.

But what can you do when you just feel really down on yourself? When you look in the mirror and really hate what you see there, and all it does is make you want to do the opposite of what you should? When your weight is affecting your self-esteem?

Well, you've already taken one of the biggest steps. You've purchased this book. You're reading it. That means you're already determined to make a change. And taking action is always a positive feeling. And on the real … the secret to self-esteem is loving yourself exactly as you are—extra pounds and all. Look at it this way—if you can love yourself even when you're not totally happy with the way you look, think of how unstoppable you'll be by the time you're pleased with your body!

You are worthy! You are a great human being with lots to offer the world. You are worthy now—not when you lose weight and not when you achieve any other goal you have. You are worthy NOW, exactly as you are." If you need to, repeat this to yourself every morning until you feel it. This is called a "positive self-affirmation." It will probably feel silly at first, but think about how often we tell ourselves something negative. If we do that enough, we'll start to believe it. So try it with something positive instead!

Don't get me wrong: learning to love yourself, especially when you are dissatisfied with your body, is hard work. Truly. But if you can't love yourself, you may never get the results you're looking for. As the cliché goes, change must start from within.

I hope you keep the lessons you learned in this chapter very close as you progress in your weight loss journey. Set the intention to approach the 1200-calorie diet from a position of peace and self-love. You are so worth it!

Chapter 2

Just the Facts, Ma'am!

O kay, so let's get down to the meat and potatoes (pardon my pun). What is the 1200-calorie diet? Well, it's just what it sounds like—a diet that limits food intake to just 1200 calories a day (Again, use 1500 as a guideline if you're a man). Unlike other diets such as Atkins and Paleo, the 1200-calorie diet doesn't eliminate entire food groups. The only requirement is to keep your calorie count to 1200 calories a day. If that sounds pretty simple, it is, in theory. You can just close this book and get started! But wait, not so fast. The rule is simple, but that doesn't mean it will be easy to implement. So there are things you should know to ensure the best results. This chapter will break down exactly how the 1200-calorie diet works.

Terms You Should Know

Let's start with some weight loss terms you'll want to be familiar with: **Body Mass Index, Metabolism, Basil Metabolic Rate**, and **Calorie.** We'll take them one at a time.

Body Mass Index

Can you just jump in and get started? Sure, but first it's a good idea to know where you stand. That means knowing your Body Mass Index (BMI). To calculate BMI, take your weight and divide it by your height. This measurement basically determines if you are at a healthy weight for your height. It reveals whether you are considered obese or are at a normal weight. It's also an indication of the degree of your health risk, if any. The higher your BMI, the more at risk you are for various diseases.

By the way, for the convenience of my print and audiobook audience, all links are available at 1200caloriediet.net/book-links. Got it? Ok. I want you to stop right now and use the BMI Calculator (at link above) to calculate your Body Mass Index. You need only your height and weight to do the calculation.

I've also created a free worksheet for you to record various details as you embark on your weight loss journey. You can find that at 1200caloriediet.net/downloads. Now go ahead and use the worksheet to record your BMI. Here's a handy chart to help evaluate where you stand. Keep in mind BMI is merely a measure of your weight against your height. It often doesn't take into account other metrics, such as how much of your weight is muscle versus fat.

BMI	CLASSIFICATION
< 18.5	Underweight
18.5–24.9	Normal Weight
25.0–29.9	Overweight
30.0+	Obesity
40.0+	Extreme Obesity

Ok, so calculating your BMI probably confirmed something you already knew—you're overweight. (If you're not, what are you doing here?) It's no fun having bad news confirmed, but that's why you're here now—to identify the problem and come up with a solution. Knowing where you stand is half the battle. Your goal is to get your weight down to the normal range, and now that you know your BMI, you can determine when you've succeeded.

Now if you're relatively fit and just trying to lose two pounds to get into the dress you wore to your high school prom, you are dismissed. Seriously, put this book down and slowly back away! Do not pass go; do not collect $200! Some of us have real problems! ☺ But all jokes aside, if you calculated your BMI and it fell within the normal range, this book likely isn't for you. The 1200-calorie diet works best for people who have a lot of weight to lose. And the more overweight you are, the more effective the results will be. So now you've been warned.

Metabolism

Metabolism refers to a process whereby the body breaks down food into small pieces. It then either turns them into energy or stores them for later. Metabolism varies from one person to another based on health, activity level, age, and other factors, and its speed determines how fast or how slowly you will lose weight. If your metabolism is slow, you'll lose weight slowly or not at all. If your metabolism is fast, you'll lose weight more quickly. Things like exercise and strength training can speed up your metabolism. The good news is there are ways to increase a slow metabolism, which we'll discuss later.

Basal Metabolic Rate

Your Basal Metabolic Rate (BMR) refers to the number of calories your body needs just to exist. It determines your body's minimum energy expenditure while at rest and how much food you require to sustain that energy expenditure. In other words, when you're just going about your normal day, how much energy does your body use? How many calories do you burn? That's BMR. Even when you are inactive, your body still needs energy to keep things running—to keep your heart beating, your lungs breathing, and your brain thinking its wise thoughts.

So yes, your body is always burning calories, even when doing things we think of as sedentary, such as watching TV, eating (yep, you burn calories while eating….fancy that!), and even sleeping. BMR tells you how many calories your body needs each day to perform these mundane, everyday activities. It varies from person to person, even between two people who otherwise have the same characteristics.

BMR is calculated using your gender, age, height, weight, and activity level. Stop right now and use this BMR Calculator (https://1200caloriediet.net/book-links/), and then record your results on the free worksheet (https://1200caloriediet.net/downloads/). You did download it, right?

In addition, here's a chart that provides pretty good estimates:

Recommended Calorie Intake				
	Men		Women	
	Activity Level		Activity Level	
Age	Sedentary	Moderate	Sedentary	Moderate
16 – 18	2400	2800	1800	2000
19 – 20	2600	2800	2000	2200
21 – 25	2400	2800	2000	2000
26 – 40	2400	2600	1800	2000
41 – 45	2200	2600	1800	2000
46 – 50	2200	2400	1800	2000
51 – 60	2200	2400	1600	1800
61 – 65	2000	2400	1600	1800
Age 66 and up	2000	2200	1600	1800

Your BMR is VERY important when you're trying to lose weight. Suppose you're a woman who weighs 170 pounds and requires 2000 calories per day for daily body maintenance. In other words, you require 2000 calories to fuel your body in its daily activities because you burn 2000 calories on a daily basis. Therefore, you should be able to eat 2000 calories and *maintain* your weight, *without exercise.* 2000 calories in and 2000 out creates a balance where you will neither lose nor gain any extra pounds. Now if you want to gain weight, you'd eat a little more than 2000 calories each day. And if you want to lose weight, you guessed it, you've got to eat less than 2000 calories.

Calorie

Here we go. This is the term you are most familiar with, and it is the nitty-gritty of weight loss. It all boils down to Calories In vs. Calories Out. I'll repeat this throughout because it's very important. And it's so simple that people complicate it unnecessarily. A calorie is a unit that measures energy. When we speak of the number of calories in food, we're referring to how much energy they provide to the body. Maintaining a healthy weight requires a balance of energy—consuming x number of calories and burning that same amount. The more calories you consume, the more energy is stored in your body. And excess energy is stored as fat, causing you to gain weight.

All foods supply energy, but nutritional value varies. Many people eat more calories than necessary but still fail to meet the recommended nutrient intake. Foods that supply only energy and no nutritional value are said to contain empty calories. They lack the daily vitamins, minerals, fiber, and other nutrients your body needs to sustain itself from day to day. They are higher in calories and often consumed in higher doses than healthier foods energy. Empty calories consist of all the things we know and love (and want more of): soda, ice cream, cookies, cake, candy, pastries, butter, alcohol, chips, fast food, etc.

When we're young, we require fewer calories to sustain our daily activities. We need more as we settle into adulthood, and our calorie needs begin to decrease again as we continue to age. In general, a male between the ages of 19 and 50 requires about 2500 calories, with that number decreasing as he ages. A woman in the same age group requires about 2000 calories. If you are overweight, it's probably because you've been consuming more calories than your body actually needs to function on a daily basis. This is why the primary way to lose weight is to burn more calories than you consume or to eat fewer calories.

1200 Calories?

So why is 1200 calories the magic number? That's considered the minimum the average body needs to function (of course, you can go lower and be fine, but only for a little while, and you should only do so if doctor-recommended). 1200 calories can provide all the nutrients you need while still promoting substantial weight loss. But it's just a guideline, a place to begin. You might find that you require slightly more calories to function. Start at 1200 and make adjustments as necessary based on how your body responds. If you're hungry all the time, increase your calorie intake by one or two hundred. You'll still be at a calorie deficit; therefore, you'll still lose weight. But give 1200 calories a fighting chance first before you decide you can't handle it. Man (Woman) Up! :-)

Seriously though, if you feel at all unwell while following the 1200-calorie diet, raise your daily calorie count. Slowing down your weight loss is preferable to not feeling your best. In addition, if you already have dietary restrictions, are pregnant, or have health issues like diabetes, high blood pressure, or heart disease, consult your doctor to determine if the 1200-calorie diet is safe for you.

Why It Works

Yep, I've got to keep saying this: The key component of weight loss is that you must create a calorie deficit—either by consuming fewer calories than your body needs or burning off extra calories through activity and exercise. The

1200-calorie diet focuses on the first part—consuming fewer calories than your body needs. It works because by staying at 1200 calories, you're automatically giving your body substantially fewer calories than it needs to sustain itself. Various diets exist, all with different names, but they all operate on this same principle in one way or another— they restrict calories. For example, people lose weight on a no-carb diet not just because they've eliminated carbs but because by eliminating carbs, they've automatically restricted their calorie intake.

If you don't get anything else from this book, please hear me on this:

For the purpose of weight loss, a calorie is a calorie. It doesn't matter if the calories come from carbs, proteins, or fats.

All of it can be stored as excess energy if you consume too much. Other things matter for overall health and nutrition, but for weight loss, it really is as simple (and hard) as that.

Here's another public service announcement: Weight loss takes work. It costs something … whether that something is less food or more exercise, it costs. No pill can make you lose weight while you sleep. No super foods can melt away fat. No cream can magically make cellulite disappear. Diets that eliminate or severely restrict entire food groups are unreasonable and hard to follow, and they cause nutritional deficiencies. You're looking for something that will help you lose weight and keep it off, right? Ok then. Enough of the yo-yo dieting! The 1200-calorie diet works because it's reasonable. It directly addresses the real problem: excess calories. It works because you can use it to lose weight safely and effectively. And when you come off of it, you can increase your calorie intake to maintenance level and keep the weight off simply by not overeating.

Now, this is not to say you can't incorporate some aspects of these other diets if they appeal to you. If you want to do low-carb, go for it. If you want to just drink a smoothie for breakfast, that's fine too. Weight Watchers and other such programs have prepackaged foods that are often low in calories, so if you like those, have one for lunch, dinner, or whenever. Just remember that whatever you decide to do, it's all about your calories at the end of the day.

Let's Talk About Pounds

When we discuss weight, we speak in pounds. We say, *I weigh 150 pounds, I weigh 200 pounds, I weigh 125 pounds (and everyone hates me)*, etc. So it helps to understand the concept of pounds and their relationship to calories when we want to lose weight. One pound of fat equals 3500 calories. That means if you want to lose one pound, you need a deficit of 3500 calories per week (About 500 calories a day). To lose two pounds a week, you need a deficit of 7000 calories over the course of a week (or 1000 calories a day). Sound impossible? It's not. On an average 2000-calorie diet, you consume 14,000 calories a week (and even more if you're prone to overeating). Looking at it from that point of view, you can see that you do have some room to limit your calories substantially each week. This is ridiculously easy on the 1200-calorie diet. Check this out:

- Suppose your calorie maintenance level (BMR) is 2000.

- Now you've decreased your calorie intake from 2000 to 1200.
- That's an 800-calorie deficit per day (2000 - 1200).
- There are 7 days in a week: 800 X 7 equals 5600 calories.
- So you've created a 5600-calorie deficit per week.
- Remember, you only need a 3500-calorie deficit to lose one pound a week or 7000 to lose two pounds a week.
- At a 5600-calorie deficit, you're losing almost two pounds a week!

I can't say it enough. This kind of calorie deficit is all you need to lose weight. No more, no less. Don't let anyone fool you into complicated gadgets and plans.

Got it? Good. Onward!

Chapter 3

Let's Get This Party Started

Now that you understand the effect of limiting your food intake to 1200 calories a day, you're ready to get started. But what's the best way to begin? The most successful goals always involve a plan for carrying them out, and weight loss is no different. Before diving headfirst into the 1200-calorie diet, you'll want to do some preparatory work. Here are the steps you will take:

1. Record your starting weight
2. Evaluate your current caloric intake
3. Determine your weight loss goal
4. Count your calories and plan your meals
5. Use a fitness tracker
6. Weigh yourself once a week
7. Take your measurements
8. Rinse and repeat …. and adjust as needed

You'll record a lot of this data on the free worksheet, so be sure to have it handy. Now let's get into each step!

Step One: Record Your Starting Weight

If you don't have a scale, you'll want to buy one because you'll be weighing yourself a lot. But for now, just find a scale anywhere to get your current weight. If you've got a Publix nearby, all of them have scales. You need to know your weight so you can determine how much you actually want to lose. To avoid unrealistic expectations, just decide how much you want to lose over the next 30 days. It's better to have several small goals rather than a long one that drags on and on.

Step Two: Evaluate Your Current Caloric Intake

Normally, the point of this step is to determine your current calorie consumption so you can figure out how much you need to reduce it to lose weight. In this case, you already know you're going down to 1200 calories, but this step is still beneficial for a few reasons:

- It's good to know your current caloric intake. Has it been terrible, a little excessive, fairly normal? You need this information to do a reality check and see how much of a change you'll need to make. The numbers will help you see how and why you gained weight. You won't be on the 1200-calorie forever, and this knowledge is the key to keeping the weight off once you start eating normally again.

- Your results on the 1200-calorie diet are directly related to the calories you currently consume. To use what I hope is an excessive example, if you currently eat 4000 calories a day and suddenly go down to 1200 calories, weight loss will come very quickly. If you've already been dieting, you might only be eating 1800, so the weight loss won't be as drastic, but it will still come. Knowing your current intake will give you an idea of the degree of weight loss you can expect and how fast when you drop down to 1200 calories.

- If you've been eating a lot, you may need to gradually decrease to 1200 calories. A sudden drop from 4000 calories to 1200 calories might be too drastic. And you might be too hungry to concentrate on the goal. Keep in mind that you will lose weight when you begin to restrict calories, even if it's not as low as 1200. You may need to pace yourself so that extreme hunger doesn't cause you to fail before you even get started. You'll lose weight more slowly, but the most important thing is that you'll still lose it. For example, dropping from 3000 calories a day to 2000 calories will still cause you to lose weight.

- If you've been trying to lose weight for a while, it's even possible that your calorie restriction may already be too low, already under 1200 calories. If so, you'll need to make adjustments to meet the 1200-calorie minimum. Consuming under 1200 calories is fine for a limited time. You might decide to fast for a few days, but don't consume beneath that number for an extended time, as that can cause your metabolism to slow down and hold on to weight instead of letting it go.

To evaluate your current calorie consumption, just eat as you normally would for a week and record the results. You can use a pen and paper, but I recommend an app like MyFitnessPal to look up calorie content and record the results.

Step Three: Determine Your Weight Loss Goal

You already know your calorie goal: 1200 per day. Now you need to set your weight loss goal. Setting a goal is important because you need a way to determine whether you're succeeding. At this point, you should know your current weight and what your healthy weight should be based on the BMI calculation. If you don't have that information yet, take a moment to go back to the BMI section and do it now. Done? Great!

Now, maybe you've determined you need to lose 50 or even 100 pounds to be within normal weight range. But should that be your immediate weight loss goal? I don't think so! There's a psychological behavioral concept ironically called "shaping," though the concept has nothing to do with fitness. The idea is that a series of small, achievable goals get you closer to the ultimate goal. Don't set your initial goal for 50 pounds. Set it for 10, or even 5. Each time you reach the smaller goal, you'll be more motivated to continue to move toward the bigger goal.

Another component of shaping is to reward yourself each time you are successful. Since you're trying to change your relationship with food, avoid using food as a reward. Reward yourself with something simple like that new CD you've been wanting or something as extravagant as a cruise.

I initially wanted to lose 30 pounds, but my initial goal was only to lose 10 pounds. I did that. Then I set my next goal to lose 10 more. I did that too. If I had started with a goal of losing 30 pounds all at once, I would have gotten discouraged by the process. But meeting those smaller goals felt great! Setting and meeting those smaller goals will feel like success because that's exactly what it is.

Here's what I did—I reached one goal and then I took a break. Sometimes it was a couple of weeks; other times it was a month, but I made sure I didn't gain any weight in my off time. I still counted calories. When my break was over, I resumed the 1200-calorie diet until the next target was reached. That was my process, but it doesn't have to be yours. You may not want to take any breaks. If I hadn't, I would likely have lost more weight in a shorter period. But I needed breaks from the diet to avoid getting burned out on it.

You should do whatever works for you, but try not to set a goal that's too high. If you have 50 pounds or less to lose, divide that goal in half and set two goals. If you have 100 pounds or more to lose, divide that goal into three or more smaller goals. Even losing 5 to 10 percent of your body weight will be a big improvement both for your health and for your body image.

So how much are you going to try to lose initially? Once you decide, write that number on your worksheet.

Step Four: Count Your Calories and Plan Your Meals

This is a crucial step to ensure you'll be able to stick to the plan. You must begin to check the calorie content of all foods. Yeah. All of them. No guesstimating! 1200 calories can add up fast, so it's essential to plan; otherwise, you'll consume too many calories before you even begin to start recording them. So what kind of food should/can you eat? I'm going to give you the politically correct *and* the politically incorrect answer.

The Politically Correct Answer: You should eat a balanced meal, which consists of 45–65% carbohydrates, 10–35% protein, and 20–35% fats, with no more than 10% saturated fats. What does that look like on a 1200-calorie diet? Your daily intake would consist of approximately 660 calories from carbohydrates, 180 calories from protein, and 360 calories from fat.

The Politically Incorrect Answer: Eat what you want, as long as at the end of the day you have consumed 1200 calories. Yep, I said it. Eat what you want, at least initially. Here's why: This diet is unlikely to be easy. If you simultaneously restrict yourself to 1200 calories and also begin a strictly "healthy" diet that you aren't used to, it can backfire. If you change too much at once, you *will* feel deprived, begin craving the good stuff, and the diet won't last long.

Now, obviously, eating anything you want isn't a long-term solution. You want to begin eating healthy to give your body the nutrients it needs. But no one said you have to do everything at once. Focus on one thing at a time and gradually begin to change your diet. Feeling deprived leads to binge eating and falling off the wagon. If you know you can still have a cheeseburger, you're more likely to stick to the diet.

Now of course, this does NOT mean you should have McDonald's for breakfast, lunch, and dinner (unless you're choosing the healthier options). You're on a restricted diet, and you do need some real nourishment and nutrition. You need to keep up your strength to avoid feeling tired all the time. You want to be able to concentrate at work and during other important tasks. Consuming 500 calories of cookies will have a different effect on your body than 500 calories of fresh vegetables. And the vegetables are better, but you already know that.

So don't take what I'm saying as an excuse to live on a steady diet of junk food. I'm saying you can keep eating what you like *in moderation*. Fortunately, the 1200-calorie diet will help with the moderation part; there's only so much wiggle room on that kind of caloric restriction. If you're already eating right, don't stop. Keep at it. But if you're not, you probably need a grace period before you're a lean, mean veggie-eating machine.

Tips For Dieting Success

My diet consisted of a mixture of healthy eating and delicious eating: sometimes I ate what I wanted; sometimes I ate healthy. Many times, I sensibly had oatmeal for breakfast, tuna for lunch, and a salad and baked fish for dinner, with room to spare for a light snack. Other times I ate no breakfast and had Kentucky Fried Chicken for lunch. I couldn't get the whole value meal I was accustomed to, but I could eat two pieces of chicken AND a biscuit and still have room for a decent-sized dinner. I couldn't get the Dave's Double from Wendy's that I absolutely loved (unless that's all I'm eating for the day), but I could certainly handle a single burger with cheese (occasionally I ate it without the bread if I needed to save calories). Leave room in your schedule to eat what you enjoy and you will be more successful. But moderation is the key. Pay attention to serving size and cut it in half if the caloric intake for the full serving is too ridiculous.

Now, I was often an angel during the week but didn't restrict myself to 1200 calories on the weekends.

I might decide to eat 2000 calories on Saturday or Sunday (sometimes both!), but on Monday, I returned to 1200 calories.

Yes. Cheat!! It will help you stick with the diet, but don't do it for more than a day or two.

Beware of Empty Calories

We discussed this earlier. Empty calories are calories that come from foods and drinks that provide little or no nutritional value. Yet they just so happen to be the kinds of foods we eat in abundance, which typically leads to weight gain.

Examples of foods with empty calories include the following:

1. **Sugary Drinks** – Soda, energy drinks, fruit-flavored drinks, and sweet coffee beverages

2. **Processed Snacks** – Chips, cookies, cakes, candy, and pastries

3. **Fast Food & Fried Foods** – French fries, fried chicken, and fast-food in general

4. **Alcohol** – Beer, wine, and spirits

5. **Certain Condiments** – Syrups, some salad dressings, and mayonnaise

Keep in mind you can eat some of these things because you're focusing on limiting your calories to 1200. However, filling up on appetite-suppressing foods will help you be more successful in sticking to this diet. You want to focus on foods like protein, fiber, dark chocolate, and spices. They will help you feel fuller without having to eat more calories. Let's take a deeper dive into each one.

Protein and Fats

One way to help you stay fuller for longer is to focus on eating enough protein and healthy fats. Compared to carbohydrates (sugars), protein and fats provide you with more energy that will sustain your body for a longer period of time. I know it sounds weird to prioritize fats to lose weight, but fats are a necessary component of your diet. Choosing to eat healthy fats and proteins is a great way to suppress your appetite. Examples of these foods include lean meats like fish and turkey, eggs, beans and lentils, Greek yogurt, nuts, avocados, and products made with soy, like tofu.

Fiber

Another way to decrease your appetite is to opt for high-fiber foods. Fiber is much slower to break down than other substances, so it stays in your body longer, increasing the time it takes for food to digest. This extended period of digestion keeps you fuller for longer. Healthy foods that are high in fiber include whole-grain bread and pasta, apples, vegetables, and avocados.

Dark Chocolate

I've got some good news for the chocolate-lovers out there! Though I don't recommend indulging too much in milk chocolate, dark chocolate has been shown to be an appetite suppressant. Obviously, don't go overboard, but a small piece of dark chocolate after a meal may help you ward off future cravings.

Spices

Spices typically have little or no calories, so you can use these to enhance your taste buds and feel more satisfied. Whether sweet or spicy, you can experiment with different spices—things like ginger and cayenne. Similarly, switching from that daily sugar in your tea to honey may also help suppress your appetite.

Beware of Liquid Calories

Because your calories are restricted, you don't want to waste them. And liquid calories can really add up. This includes soda, Kool-Aid, punch, sweet tea (my personal weakness), and even fruit juices. The average regular-size drink will run you 200 to 300 calories. The question you've got to ask yourself is, "Do I really want to spend X calories on this drink?" Some days the answer might be yes; other times it might be no. But those are the kinds of decisions you'll have to make. For the most part, I cut out sodas and other drinks (except on the weekends) and stuck primarily to water. I didn't want to waste my calories on them. I wanted to eat!

Beware of Sauces, Condiments, and Dressings

Remember, you must count calories for even the smallest thing, and that includes items you put on your food, like mayo, butter, sour cream, and salad dressing. These things can easily add 100 calories or more to a meal. Again, I'm not saying you have to totally eliminate them; I'm saying know what you're eating at all times. Now if you opt for the low-fat versions of these items, you can cut down considerably on the calories.

Beware of Food Nutrition Labels

The food industry uses a standard Nutrition Facts label on all foods to allow you to evaluate the nutritional content. It provides information regarding serving size, calories, nutrients, and sometimes recommended dietary guidelines based on a 2000- or 2500-calorie diet. This should be very helpful in your journey to weight loss. Unfortunately, many of the labels can be misleading. They aren't that straightforward about how many calories you may actually be consuming. Many foods that are typically consumed as a package often contain more than one serving. So when you're evaluating a label for calories, pay special attention to these three lines, which are normally somewhere near the top:

- Serving Size
- Servings Per Container
- Amount Per Serving or Calories Per Serving

Sample Label for
Macaroni and Cheese

Nutrition Facts

Serving Size 1 cup (228g)
Servings Per Container 2

Amount Per Serving

Calories 250	Calories from Fat 110

	% Daily Value*
Total Fat 12g	18%
Saturated Fat 3g	15%
Trans Fat 1.5g	
Cholesterol 30mg	10%
Sodium 470mg	20%
Total Carbohydrate 31g	10%
Dietary Fiber 0g	0%
Sugars 5g	
Protein 5g	

Vitamin A	4%
Vitamin C	2%
Calcium	20%
Iron	4%

* Percent Daily Values are based on a 2,000 calorie diet.
Your Daily Values may be higher or lower depending on
your calorie needs:

	Calories:	2,000	2,500
Total Fat	Less than	65g	80g
Sat Fat	Less than	20g	25g
Cholesterol	Less than	300mg	300mg
Sodium	Less than	2,400mg	2,400mg
Total Carbohydrate		300g	375g
Dietary Fiber		25g	30g

Here's how they all interact: First, the package will tell you what measurement constitutes a serving size. It may be 1 cup, 5 cookies, 20 chips, etc. Servings per container tells you how many servings are in the package. So there may be 5 cookies in a serving but 3 servings in the package. Finally, the calories per serving tells you how many calories are in *one* serving, not in the whole package—just in that one serving. If you look at the calorie line and conclude that number refers to the whole container, you'll often be incorrect. One benefit to eating out is that the calories listed often refer to the whole item rather than just part of it. But let's look at some real-life examples:

Now with some things, what you see is what you get. The calorie content is very clear, for example, with many brands of tuna. The serving size is often one can, so you know exactly how many calories you'll eat if you consume the whole can.

But here's a perfect example of what I call deceitful food labels: Nabisco makes these delicious snack bags of mini Oreo cookies (my weakness). The serving size is 9 cookies and the calories per serving is 140. But here's the catch—there are *three* servings in the bag. So if I eat the entire bag, I'm not eating 140 calories—I'm eating 420. That's a big difference! You can imagine how much that kind of mistake will cost you if that's your favorite snack and you think it's only 140 calories.

Here's another example where it seems the food label is setting me up to fail (but it can't because I'm on to it). Walmart has these delicious pork chops stuffed with bacon and cheese. There are two pre-seasoned pieces in the pack, and all you do is transfer the meat to a pan and bake it. But here's the catch: the nutrition label says the calorie count is 300. My logical mind says, "Oh, each pork chop is 300 calories." But that isn't the case. Why? Because of the serving size. Each serving is *half a pork chop*, not a full one. So a full pork chop is 600 calories. Seriously, why all the shenanigans? Why not just list the calories per pork chop? But companies do this with their food labels all the time to make the calorie content seem lower.

You're going to be smarter than them, though. Just remember that the calorie count you initially see always refers to the serving size, and always know exactly how many servings are in the container you are consuming.

Beware of Restaurants

Restaurants are not your friend unless you eat VERY consciously. You can easily consume 4000 to 5000 calories in one meal between the entrée, appetizer, and constant drink refills. It's fine to treat yourself, but make sure you know the caloric intake before you order anything. Even some salads are often 1000 calories! I can't stress it enough. Even if you think something is healthy, look up the calorie content! Nowadays, many restaurants have calorie info on their menu, but if not, just ask Google, an AI chatbot, or look up the info on the company's website.

Get used to checking calories *before* you eat any meal, preferably before you even leave the house. Decide what you're going to have before you even get there. Don't wait until after you've eaten to find that you've gone way over your quota and now you can't eat for the rest of the week! :-) Remember this: If it's fried, sauced, creamy, or cheesy, it's high in calories. You may still be able to eat it by consuming only half, or even a third. But know what you're eating.

Tips for Eating Out

- Ask for a to-go box and immediately split your meal in half. To-go boxes will definitely be your friend since restaurant portions are often large. You don't have to eat everything in front of you.

- Share your meal with your dinner date. Many times, the entrees or appetizers are so big that you can just order one.
- Eat your salad first, though you still need to check the calorie content. It's full of nutrients and fiber that will keep you feeling full, but it's lower in calories. You likely won't be able to eat all of your entrée when it comes, and that's a good thing.
- Order an appetizer and skip the full meal altogether. Eating a whole appetizer plus the entrée will pile on the calories.
- Have sauces, gravies, and dressings brought to you on the side so you can decide how much to use.
- Drink water or unsweetened tea to cut down on the empty calories we so often get from drinks.
- Avoid buffets unless you can be very, VERY disciplined. (It's better to save buffets for your cheat day anyway). Piling your plate at such establishments is just too tempting, even if you tell yourself you're only going to have a little taste of everything.

- Skip dessert unless you have purposely saved the calories for it ahead of time. But it's safer to opt for low-calorie sweets such as fruit, JELL-O, or pudding.
- Eat until you feel satisfied, and then stop. You're not a kid anymore, so you don't have to abide by the "clean-your-plate" rule.
- Order substitutes when opting for fast food: a potato or salad instead of fries; pizza with vegetable toppings instead of meat; burgers without cheese or bread; grilled chicken instead of breaded, and small fries and drink instead of large.
- Don't make assumptions. For example, it sounds reasonable to order a chicken sandwich instead of a burger. We just have it in our heads as a society that chicken is healthier. But if the chicken is fried or breaded instead of grilled, the hamburger is often the lower-calorie option.

Weekly Calorie Intake Versus Daily Intake

It may help to think in terms of weekly caloric intake instead of daily caloric intake, as it gives you more wiggle room. 1200 calories a day equals 8400 calories a week. Let's say you cheat one Monday and eat 1800 calories. You would simply adjust accordingly throughout the week to ensure ending the week with a total of 8400 calories. Of course, you can subtract that extra 600 the next day and only eat 600 calories, but a better plan is to spread it over the next six days. So you'd eat 1100 calories each day instead of 1200.

And if at the end of one week you find that you actually ate 9000 calories instead of 8400, don't sweat it. You're still at a significant calorie deficit and you'll still lose weight. Just don't make a habit of going over. You'll want to stay at 8400 calories per week to get the most out of the 1200-calorie diet, but don't panic if you occasionally eat a little more.

You Can Ignore These Common Dieting Rules

If I had a dollar for all the fake dieting rules that exist, I'd be a millionaire! You can safely ignore all of these because your rule is very simple: Eat 1200 calories a day.

Eat Six Small Meals a Day

Some people say you should eat six small meals a day because it speeds up your metabolism. But studies have shown that's not necessarily true. The most important thing is to eat in such a way that you will stick to your goal. Your goal is 1200 calories a day, so what's the best way for YOU to reach that goal without feeling too tired or too hungry or too grumpy or too deprived? It's up to you.

The only reason to eat six small meals is to avoid feeling hungry and overeating. That's it. But you might be like me and find it inconvenient to eat that many meals. Plus, dividing your meals like that on a 1200-calorie diet will result in a bunch of small, unsatisfying meals. Each meal would have to be around 200 calories! To me, that's no fun at all. I prefer to save my calories so I can have three satisfying meals, or two really satisfying meals and a snack.

Always Eat Breakfast

Breakfast is the most important meal of the day, they say. Don't ever skip it, they say. But maybe you're like me and you're not really a breakfast person. Don't force yourself. Feel free to skip it and save those calories to eat more at lunch or dinner, or for that snack you know you'll need later in the evening. If you want breakfast, eat it. If you don't, skip it.

Don't Eat Dinner After a Certain Time

Some "experts" claim that if you eat carbs in the evening or eat dinner after a certain time, you will gain weight. But as long as you stay in a calorie deficit, like you will on the 1200-calorie diet, you could eat at midnight and still lose weight. The calories you eat at noon are the same calories you eat at midnight. Yes, really! A calorie is a calorie is a calorie. Calories don't suddenly change and add more pounds because of the time of day or the type of food.

Now, it's true that eating late can be problematic, but only because people who tend to have late-night cravings end up eating extra calories. People who gain weight like this have already eaten their calorie quota for the day, and now around 10 p.m., they're devouring an extra bag of chips or a whole pack of cookies.

Those extra snacks will certainly add to the overall calorie count. But you're not going to eat like that—not at 10 p.m. and not at 10 a.m. either. You've got a calorie goal to meet. See the difference? It's not the time of day or type of calorie that causes you to gain weight—it's the excess consumption of those calories. So just know that it isn't the act of eating late that causes a person to gain weight. Hit your caloric goal on whatever schedule works best for you.

You Have to Starve Yourself

You don't have to starve yourself in order to lose weight. You don't have to feel deprived. 1200 calories might sound like you are starving yourself, but it's really not. You can actually feel pretty satisfied if you focus on eating the right combination of foods—protein, fiber, etc.

You Can't Eat Dessert or Fast Food

You've seen this in action. People find out you're on a diet and then they see you eating a piece of cake or having a mouth-watering burger. And they can't resist calling you on it—"I thought you were trying to lose weight," they'll say. They don't understand that you're focusing on calories over food types. Again, as long as you stay within 1200 calories, you can eat what you want!

Follow Guidelines, Not Rules

All of these rules have good intentions, and it's true that they can be helpful. If you eat smaller meals throughout the day, you will, in general, be less hungry and less likely to overeat. Same with eating breakfast. If you stay away from food late at night, you're less likely to fall victim to the eat-a-whole-bag-of-chips trap. But these are only guidelines. Don't follow rules just for the sake of following rules. Follow them if they work for you, but if they don't work or they cause stress, don't follow them.

I hope I'm being clear. Do what works for you. If eating breakfast will give you the required energy you need to wake up and feel alert, then eat breakfast. If eating breakfast will prevent you from being hungry and wolfing down a 1500-calorie cheeseburger at lunch, then yes, eat breakfast. But don't do it just to meet some arbitrary gotta-eat-breakfast rule.

What's the goal? 1200 calories a day. That's your only rule—by any means you want to accomplish it. Got it? Good.

Don't Forget the Water!

Water is essential to your overall health because it makes up over half of your body composition. You lose water on a daily basis, and that water needs to be replaced. Dehydration occurs when the water you lose exceeds the water you consume. Water depletion occurs in various ways: as perspiration through the skin, water vapor through the lungs, or urine through the kidneys. There are other ways to lose water, but those are the main pathways. Water out requires water in.

How much water you should consume depends on various factors, such as physical activity and weight. A good guideline is to consume about half your body weight in ounces. The more you weigh, the more water you'll need. If you weigh 200 pounds, you'll want to drink at least 100 ounces per day. As you lose weight, your water intake needs will decrease as well. But you'll need to drink more if you're very active.

How do you know when you've had enough water? Your urine should be nearly colorless. Yellow means drink! You should drink water continuously throughout the day, before you feel thirsty. Thirst is a sign that you're already dehydrated.

Drinking water is also helpful in your weight loss journey. It helps increase your metabolism and flush out waste products from your body, especially excess sodium that makes you feel bloated. It also acts as an appetite suppressant, which means it keeps you feeling fuller for longer and will ward off hunger pains. When your body is holding excess water weight, increasing your quota will encourage your body to eliminate it, which will lower that number on the scale.

Drinking water should be considered one of the most valuable tools in your weight-loss toolbox. Make a point to drink a big glass of water as soon as you wake up. Drink up again right before each meal. This will help fill you up so that you can eat less but still feel full. If you're trying to cut calorie-dense sodas and juice out of your diet, water is the perfect alternative. Though it may not be your favorite thing at first, you might find that you begin to prefer water to soda after a month or two. You can also add a few slices of cucumber or a lemon wedge to your water to make it taste better. Also, there are low-calorie flavored waters and plain tea if you can't stomach plain water.

Don't underestimate the importance of water in succeeding with the 1200-calorie diet.

Take a Vitamin Supplement

While eating only 1200 calories, it is possible you won't manage to get all the nutrients you need every day. If you're worried about this, take a vitamin supplement. It will give you more energy and fill in the gaps of any nutrient deficiencies.

Step Five: Use a Fitness Tracker

Many websites/apps allow you to look up the calorie content in food, input your fitness goals, and track your progress in achieving those goals. MyFitness-Pal.com is just one of the many available. There are some paid options, but don't bother with them. The free options provide tools that are more than adequate for your needs. I initially used MyFitnessPal and then graduated to using a Fitbit. But remember, you can use any tool that gets the job done. If for some reason you don't want to use MyFitnessPal, just do a quick Google for "free calorie tracker apps."

Using an app is one of the most helpful things I did. Why? Because to succeed on the 1200-calorie diet, you must log all calories, whether it's a grape or a slice of pizza, and don't forget drinks and sauces. The best method is to plan your calorie intake ahead of time. So plan the night before what you'll have for breakfast, and log it. If the app allows it, input food for the next day as well. You can plan the day before or a few hours before a meal. Planning ahead ensures there will be no surprises and that you have met your calorie goal at the end of the day.

As I stated, I now have a Fitbit, and I'd be lost without it. The Fitbit monitors everything! Heart rate. Calories expended. Steps taken. Everything. If nothing else, wearing something that constantly tells me how my day is going is one heck of a motivator. But at this point in your journey, there's no need to pay for anything. You can do that if you like when you're at a more advanced level in your fitness.

Step Six: Weigh Yourself Once a Week

For consistent results, weigh yourself once a week at the same time of day—preferably in the morning after using the restroom, before eating, and before getting dressed. That means if you don't already have one, you'll want to buy a scale. If you can't get one just yet, go to Publix once a week and weigh yourself there. Do not weigh yourself every day. I can already tell you it will be very tempting, but don't do that to yourself. Weight can fluctuate anywhere from 3 to 6 pounds in a day and doesn't always paint a true picture. This fluctuation has to do with water weight, food intake, sodium retention, and muscle gain. That's why it's important that you remain consistent with the time and day of the week you decide to weigh yourself.

Depending on a variety of factors, you can lose anywhere from two to four pounds a week, but don't panic if that's not happening. Give it some time. You might lose those pounds every two weeks or every three weeks instead of once a week. And don't forget that water weight and your monthly period can make your weight fluctuate significantly from one week to the next.

Some weeks I didn't lose any weight, and other weeks it seemed I'd gained a pound or two. Yet a month later, I'd realize I had lost several pounds. A good rule of thumb when it comes to weight fluctuations is to compare month to month. For example, you'll keep weighing yourself once a week and recording the results. But to judge your true weight loss, wait a month. Compare your weight on May 1 to your weight on June 1, for example. That will give you a truer picture than anything else. Now, if you haven't lost any weight at all after a month, which is HIGHLY unlikely on this diet, turn to Chapter Five for possible solutions.

If you're likely to feel frustrated due to slow weight loss, choose to weigh yourself monthly instead. On a monthly basis, you're more likely to notice major changes in your weight. And remember to be kind to yourself! There's no need to stress out over the number on the scale every week if you don't have to. That being said, I think you'll like the week-to-week results, at least initially.

Step Seven: Take Your Measurements

In many cases, the scale doesn't tell the whole story. If you haven't seen the number on the scale change in a while even though you've been doing your best, don't worry! You'll see a more complete picture of your progress if you also keep track of your body measurements.

All you'll need is a cloth measuring tape or a tape specifically designed to take body measurements. When you measure yourself, either wear tight-fitting clothing or nothing at all. Be sure to wear the same thing every time to ensure your numbers remain consistent. Similarly, take your measurements at the same time to account for daily weight fluctuations. It's best to do this in the morning before you've had anything to eat or drink, but it's more important to choose a time that fits your schedule. To increase accuracy, try taking at least two measurements for each area of the body and then recording the average.

Use the free worksheet to record your measurements. There are seven areas of the body that you may want to keep track of.

1. **Waist**: Wrap the tape around the narrowest part of your torso.

2. **Hips**: Measure at the widest part of your hips and glutes. Keep the tape parallel to the floor.

3. **Chest**: With your feet together and your back straight, wrap the tape around the widest part of your chest.

4. **Abs**: Stand tall with your feet together and measure the widest section of your torso, which is usually around your belly button.

5. **Arms**: Relax your arm and measure the halfway point between your shoulder and elbow. Repeat for the other arm.

6. **Thighs**: Measure the widest part of the thigh, or the midpoint between the bottom of your buttocks and the back of your knee. Repeat for the other leg.

7. **Calves**. Measure the midpoint between your knee and your ankle. Repeat for the other leg.

Repeat this process every month to gauge your progress. If you find that you're losing inches but maintaining weight, then you've likely gained muscle. Congratulate yourself on making great progress! If both your measurements and the scale suggest that your body isn't changing, try not to be too hard on yourself. Later, I'm going to give you some strategies to follow if you're not seeing the desired results.

Step Eight: Rinse and Repeat … and Adjust as Needed

You're in this for the long haul, until you reach your goal weight. When you reach it, pat yourself on the back, take a short break if you want, or set a new goal weight and keep on truckin'.

Initially, you will lose weight fast … very fast. And you'll be thrilled. I know I was! I think I lost the first 10 pounds in two weeks! And yeah, yeah, yeah, it won't all be fat—a lot of it will be water weight—but that doesn't stop the weight loss from being immensely satisfying. But after the initial reduction in pounds, you will progress more slowly. If you know what to expect, then you won't be surprised when that slowdown happens. And if the weight loss slows down too much, there are ways to speed it up again. We'll cover that later.

Making Adjustments to the 1200-Calorie Diet

Don't be afraid to make adjustments. Have you given it a month but you're getting too hungry on 1200 calories? Try eating slower to allow your brain to register that your hunger is satisfied. Drink water before meals. Eat lots of vegetables and fruits and fill up on fiber and protein. But if none of that helps and you need to eat a little more, do it. Also, don't continue the diet if it's making you sick, fatigued, dizzy, or has any other negative side effects. If you didn't go see your doctor before you started, stop the diet and go see him now. He may put you on a different diet based on your health needs. You want to lose weight, not die trying. So don't ignore signs that the diet isn't working for you.

Chapter 4

Let's Talk About the FOOD!

O h, hello there! I didn't see you for a second. Since you're still here, I guess we need to actually talk about the food? Initially, I really wasn't going to include this section because your food consumption only has one rule. I'll say it one more time for the people in the back: Keep your calorie intake at 1200 calories.

As I stated earlier, I didn't follow any meal plans. Instead, I simply started checking the caloric composition of my favorite foods. It really is that simple. You might call this the *Eat Anything You Want* plan. Choose your food for the day, and then just keep it at 1200. But for those of you who need a little more structure, I get it. Some of you just reeeeaaaaallly need more information on this, so let's talk about it. Now, there are countless meal plans out there, and you can find them with a simple Google search. I won't try to reproduce them here, so I'll share some links to get you started.

1200-Calorie Meal Plans

If you find it's too much of a headache to plan your own meals, you might want to follow a pre-prepared plan. There are many 1200-calorie meal plans available. Here are a few to get you started. Again, if you're reading the print book, visit 1200caloriediet.net/links for a list of these websites.

- Good Housekeeping: A 7-Day, 1,200-Calorie Weight Loss Meal Plan
- National Heart Lung and Blood Institute: Traditional American Cuisine: 1,200 Calories
- Eating Well: Simple 1200-Calorie Meal Plan

I didn't follow a meal plan because most of them contained foods I knew I'd never have time to make or foods I didn't find appetizing. So I simply accumulated a list of my favorite foods along with their calorie content. Again, there's no hard and fast rule regarding following a pre-made plan or not. Do what works.

The important thing is to plan ahead based on your eating habits and work schedule. You may need to carry snacks or bring your breakfast, lunch, or dinner with you to work. Not having a plan often leads to just grabbing calorie-filled fast food because it's convenient (and, of course, delicious). Remember, if you do visit that drive-thru, it should be because you planned it, not because it's fast and you weren't prepared.

Consider a Meal-Prep Delivery Service

I didn't know about these meal delivery services when I first did the 1200-calorie diet. But if you can afford them, they can really take the headache out of deciding what to eat. And the meals are often anywhere from 500 to 800 calories. So far, I have tried both Home Chef and Factor, and I enjoyed both. But there are so many to choose from, so just type "meal prep delivery" into Google and you'll have as many options as you can handle.

Cook at Home

Like I said before, it can seem impossible to find time to plan and cook a meal. I completely understand that. However, cooking your own food is the best way to ensure that you can control the calories you're consuming. So I recommend learning how to whip up some simple, low-calorie meals.

There are many benefits to cooking at least one meal a day. For one, you'll save money. When you go out to eat, you're not just paying for the food; you're paying for the atmosphere, food preparation, and the paychecks of the staff. When you buy food from the supermarket, you're not paying for all those extras. Another reason to cook at home is that it helps bring your family together. And it doesn't just have to be you in the kitchen! Involve your kids or your partner in the cooking process. That way, you can enjoy each other's company while also saving money and making better food choices. Finally, cooking at home naturally lowers the calories you'll consume. A meal cooked at home can contain half the calories of the same meal in a restaurant.

Become Familiar With Calories in Foods

Make no mistake, eating 1200 calories a day requires some planning. You can't just roll out of bed and start eating without giving some thought to your meals for that day. You can't eat breakfast without considering what you might have for lunch. In other words, you'll need to ask yourself this question: *If I eat ABC for breakfast or XYZ for lunch, how many calories can I eat at dinner time*?

Here is the golden rule of the 1200-calorie diet: Never eat anything without knowing how many calories it has! So you'll want to begin to learn the calorie content in various foods. How much will it cost against your bank of 1200 calories to have that soda, that hot dog, that bag of chips, that smoothie, that granola bar, that large salad?

So without further ado, let's talk about the calories in some major foods! This will be a broad overview so you can start to have an idea of calorie content as you make your decisions throughout the day. You can always use an app or the internet to find the calories for almost anything, including fast food. However, it's good to also commit some general guidelines to memory. So that's the purpose of the following charts. Note that calorie counts are subject to change, particularly with fast food items, so consider all the calorie amounts as estimates. And yes, there will inevitably be some common foods that I forgot to include. And that's ok because this list isn't meant to be exhaustive, and you can use Google to fill in the gaps.

Vegetables

Vegetables will be your best friend! Not just because they are healthy and give you most of the nutrients you need but also because veggies can be eaten in bulk without adding a ton of calories, yet they are tremendously filling. A good rule of thumb is to fill half your plate with vegetables. You almost don't need to count these calories because you are unlikely to consume enough in a day to make a big difference. However, for our purposes, you will count everything, even veggies. So here are some calorie counts:

FOOD	SERVING	CALORIES	FOOD	SERVING	CALORIES	FOOD	SERVING	CALORIES
Avocado	1 medium	240	Cucumber	1 medium	45	Peppers	1 medium	25
Beans (Other)	1 cup cooked	220	Green Peas	1 cup	62	Plantains	1 medium	220
Broccoli	1 cup chopped	55	Kale	1 cup chopped	34	Potato	1 medium (baked)	161
Carrots	1 medium	25	Lettuce	2 cups shredded	10	Spinach	1 cup raw	7
Cauliflower	1 cup chopped	27	Mushrooms	1 cup sliced	15	String Beans	1 cup cooked	31
Celery	1 cup chopped	16	Okra	1 cup sliced	33	Sweet Potato	1 medium (baked)	103
Collard Greens	1 cup chopped	11	Olives (Green)	1 cup	195	Tomato	1 medium	22
Corn	1 medium ear	77	Olives (Black)	1 cup	160	Turnip Greens	1 cup chopped	18
Corn Kernels	1 cup	132	Onions	1 medium	46	Zucchini	1 cup sliced	20

Fruit

Fruit is vegetables' kissing cousin. It's also very good for you and often low in calories, though you will have to be careful about consuming fruit juices because it's easier to drink too much and exceed your calorie goals. Fruits are excellent and often satisfying alternatives to things like cakes, cookies, muffins, candy, and all the sweet stuff we crave.

FOOD	SERVING	CALORIES	FOOD	SERVING	CALORIES
Apple	1 medium	95	Clementine	1 medium	35
Apricot	3 medium	50	Coconut	1 cup shredded	283
Banana	1 medium	105	Cranberry	1 cup	46
Blackberry	1 cup	62	Date	1 date	23
Blueberry	1 cup	84	Fig	2 medium	37
Cantaloupe	1 cup	54	Grape	1 cup	104
Cherry	1 cup	87	Grapefruit	1 medium	52

FOOD	SERVING	CALORIES	FOOD	SERVING	CALORIES
Kiwi	1 medium	61	Pear	1 medium	101
Lemon	1 medium	17	Pineapple	1 cup chunks	83
Lime	1 medium	20	Plum	2 medium	70
Mango	1 cup diced	100	Pomegranate	1 cup	83
Orange	1 medium	62	Raspberry	1 cup	64
Papaya	1 cup cubes	59	Strawberry	1 cup	50
Peach	1 medium	59	Watermelon	1 cup cubes	46

Meat and Animal Products

Most people don't know this, but protein is extremely important both for general health and for weight loss. Meat and animal products are vital sources of protein, so contrary to popular belief, you shouldn't eliminate meat just to lose weight. While you can get some protein from other sources, meat products provide it in abundance. Now if you are vegan or vegetarian, you can find good sources of protein other than meat. Some of those include eggs, nuts, beans, lentils, soy, yogurt, quinoa, tofu, green peas, oats, broccoli, spinach, asparagus, artichokes, potatoes, sweet potatoes, and Brussels sprouts.

Protein plays a role in maintaining all the cells in your body. It repairs damaged tissue and supports muscle growth. It also gives you that full feeling, whereas a lack of adequate protein can cause intense hunger. And we all know that hunger is the enemy of any weight loss program.

Animal Products

FOOD	SERVING	CALORIES
Butter	1 tablespoon	102
Cheese (American)	1 slice	70
Cheese (Provolone)	1 slice	80
Cheese (Cheddar)	1 slice	90
Cheese (Swiss)	1 slice	90
Cottage Cheese	1/2 cup	100
Eggs (Large)	1 large egg	72
Milk (Whole)	1 cup	150
Milk (2%)	1 cup	130
Milk (Skim)	1 cup	90
Ricotta Cheese	1/2 cup	200
Sour Cream	2 tablespoons	60
Yogurt (Plain)	1 cup	95
Yogurt (Sweetened)	1 cup	140

Meat and Fish

FOOD	SERVING	CALORIES	FOOD	SERVING	CALORIES	FOOD	SERVING	CALORIES
Anchovies	1 ounce	42	Chicken Thigh	1 medium-sized thigh	120	Hot Dogs (Pork)	1 hot dog	180
Bacon	2 slices	86	Chicken Wing	1 medium-sized wing	43	Hot Dogs (Turkey)	1 hot dog	100
Basa	1 fillet (6 ounces)	120	Clam Strips	3 ounces	195	Kielbasa	1 sausage	325
Beef Roast	1 medium-sized portion	160	Cornish Hen	1/2 hen (about 16 ounces)	550	Lamb	1 medium-sized portion	235
Bison	3 ounces	143	Crab (Blue)	1 medium-sized crab	82	Liver	1 slice	175
Bologna	2 slices	90	Crab Cake	1 medium-sized cake	200	Mackerel	1 fillet	231
Bratwurst	1 sausage	283	Duck	1 medium-sized portion	171	Mahi-Mahi	1 fillet	100
Calamari	3 ounces	78	Flounder	1 fillet	100	Mussels	3 ounces	146
Catfish	1 fillet (6 ounces)	105	Goat	3 ounces	122	Neck Bones	1 piece	171
Caviar	1 tablespoon	42	Grouper	1 fillet (6 ounces)	150	Oxtails	1 piece	220
Chicken (Canned)	1 can (drained)	140	Haddock	1 fillet	90	Oysters	6 medium	57
Chicken Breast	1 medium-sized breast	165	Halibut	1 fillet	120	Pastrami	3 slices	80
Chicken Breast	3 slices	60	Ham	3 slices	150	Perch	1 fillet	129
Chicken Leg	1 medium-sized leg	170	Ham Hocks	1 piece	285	Pheasant	1 bird	130
			Hot Dogs (Beef)	1 hot dog	137	Pork Chop	1 medium-sized chop	194

FOOD	SERVING	CALORIES	FOOD	SERVING	CALORIES
Pork Ribs	1 medium-sized portion	300	Snow Crab Legs	1 pound	500
Pork Roast	1 medium-sized portion	150	Steak	1 medium-sized portion	180
Quail	1 bird	150	Swordfish	1 fillet	220
Rabbit	3 oz	147	Tilapia	1 fillet	120
Roast Beef	2 slices	60	Trout	1 fillet	148
Salami	2 slices	120	Tuna	1 can	140
Salmon	1 fillet	180	Turkey (cold cut)	1 slice	30
Sardines	1 can (3.75 oz)	191	Turkey Breast	3 slices	60
Sausage (Breakfast)	2 links	170	Turkey Leg	1 leg	593
Scallops	1 large scallop (1 ounce)	25	Turkey Thigh	1 thigh	229
Short Ribs	1 medium-sized portion	300	Turkey Wing	1 wing	155
Shrimp	4 large shrimp	30	Veal	1 piece	166
Smoked Sausage (Hillshire, etc.)	Half a package	560	Venison	1 steak	150

Grains

The grains category includes rice, bread, pastries, pasta, crackers, hot cereals like oatmeal and grits, cold breakfast cereals, quinoa, and tortillas.

FOOD	SERVING	CALORIES	FOOD	SERVING	CALORIES	FOOD	SERVING	CALORIES
Apple Jacks	1 cup	110	Frosted Mini Wheats	1 cup	210	Raisin Bran Crunch	1 cup	190
Bagel	1 medium-sized bagel	245	Grits	1 cup	150	Rice (White)	1 cup cooked	205
Biscuit	1 biscuit	175	Hamburger Bun	1 medium-sized bun	120	Rice Cakes	2 rice cakes	70
Captain Crunch	1 cup	150	Hotdog Bun	1 medium-sized bun	90	Rice Krispies	1 cup	100
Cheerios	1 cup	100	Jasmine Rice	1 cup	180	Rice-A-Roni	1 cup	280
Chex Cereal	1 cup	120	Life Cereal	1 cup	120	Sliced Bread	1 slice	70-100
Cornbread	1 piece	180	Macaroni	1 cup	220	Spaghetti	1 cup	220
Cream of Wheat	1 cup cooked	133	Oatmeal	1 cup cooked	154	Special K	1 cup	120
English Muffin	1 medium-sized muffin	134	Pancakes	1 pancake	100	Tortilla	1 medium-sized tortilla	94
Froot Loops	1 cup	110	Pita	1 piece	165	Waffles	1 waffle	125
Frosted Flakes	1 cup	140	Popcorn	3 cups popped	93	Yeast Roll	1 medium-sized roll	110
			Quinoa	1 cup cooked	222	Yellow Rice	1 cup	225

Snacks and Dessert

Snacks include chips, pretzels, cookies, cake, candy, etc. You need not fear this category, or really any other categories. All you have to do is spend your calories wisely. Obviously, you don't want to snack all day, every day unless your choices are very low in calories, but you can easily work in an enjoyable snack several times a week. In fact, you should definitely do this to avoid feeling deprived. If you always remember the first rule of this diet—consume only 1200 calories—what you eat becomes a nonissue.

FOOD	SERVING	CALORIES	FOOD	SERVING	CALORIES
Apple Pie	1 slice	320	Fruit Salad	1 cup	80
Apple Sauce	1 cup	100	Honey Bun	1 bun	240
Banana Nut Bread	1 slice	200	Ice Cream	1 cup	270
Bear Claw	1 piece	400	Jello	1 cup	80
Blueberry Muffin	1 muffin	300	Oreo Cookie	2 cookies	100
Brownie	1 piece	150	Peach Cobbler	1 cup	400
Cheesecake	1 slice	300	Pecan Pie	1 slice	500
Chocolate Cake	1 slice	350	Pudding	1 cup	130
Chocolate Chip Cookie	1 cookie	50	Pumpkin Pie	1 slice	180
Coffee Cake	1 piece	200	Strawberry Shortcake	1 piece	180
Cupcake	1 cupcake	250	Sweet Potato Pie	1 slice	280
Danish	1 piece	250	Tiramisu	1 piece	200
Donut	1 glazed donut	190	Twinkie	1 cake	135

Beverages

You have to be very careful with beverages, even healthy ones like smoothies and fruit juices. I like the Spinach Pineapple smoothie from Smoothie King. It's loaded with lots of good foods and is highly nutritious. But I NEVER get a small. I always get the 32-ounce, which runs me 540 calories. On the 1200-calorie diet, that pretty much equals a whole meal. With fruit juices, you'd be fine if you kept it to 8 ounces, but I typically use an 18-ounce cup, so any juice I drink adds up to about 250 calories. In general, I prefer to eat my calories rather than drink them. And you'll likely feel more satisfied if you do the same. If you love fruit juice, you might want to buy some 8-ounce cups to make sure you don't overdo it.

FOOD	SERVING	CALORIES	FOOD	SERVING	CALORIES
Almond Milk	1 cup	60	Iced Coffee (Sweetened)	16 ounces	200
Apple Juice	1 cup	114	Iced Tea (Sweetened)	16 ounces	180
Beer (Regular)	12 ounces	150	Lemonade	1 cup	99
Black Tea	1 cup	2	Milk (Skim)	1 cup	80
Cappuccino (Starbucks)	12 ounces	60-120	Milk (2%)	1 cup	120
Caramel Frappuccino (Starbucks)	12 ounces	300	Milk (Whole)	1 cup	150
Coca Cola	1 can (12 ounces)	140	Orange Juice	1 cup	112
Coconut Water	1 cup	46	Orange Soda (Fanta)	1 can (12 ounces)	150
Coffee (Black)	1 cup	2	Pineapple Juice	1 cup	133
Coffee with Cream	1 cup	50	Red Wine	5 ounces	125
Cranberry Juice	1 cup	116	Root Beer	1 can (12 ounces)	150
Flavored Water	1 bottle (16 oz)	0-10	Smoothie (Fruit)	1 cup	120
Grape Juice	1 cup	152	Soy Milk	1 cup	100
Green Tea	1 cup	2	Sports Drink	20 ounces	140
Hawaiian Punch	1 cup	100	Sprite	1 can (12 ounces)	140
Herbal Tea	1 cup	0	Water	1 cup	0
Hot Chocolate	1 cup	192	White Wine	5 ounces	121

Condiments and Sauces

Some people make a big deal about watching this category while trying to lose weight. While caution is always a good thing, I feel this category is likely the least of your worries. For example, salad dressing will probably add more calories than anything else. But in the grand scheme of things, your salad is likely low in calories, so even if you add 100 calories with the dressing, your meal won't cost you too much. I'll keep repeating it—always know how many calories you're adding, even with sauces. Plan your meal with them in mind and you'll be just fine.

FOOD	SERVING	CALORIES		FOOD	SERVING	CALORIES		FOOD	SERVING	CALORIES
A1 Steak Sauce	1 Tbsp	15		Hot Sauce	1 Tbsp	0		Salt	1 Tsp	0
BBQ Sauce	2 Tbsp	70		Horseradish	1 Tbsp	7		Salsa	2 Tbsp	10
Basil	1 Tbsp	1		Italian Dressing	2 Tbsp	80		Seasoned Salt	1 Tsp	0
Blue Cheese Dressing	2 Tbsp	150		Ketchup	1 Tbsp	20		Sesame Seeds	1 Tbsp	52
Buffalo Sauce	2 Tbsp	20		Maple Syrup	2 Tbsp	100		Smoked Paprika	1 Tsp	6
Caesar Dressing	2 Tbsp	160		Marinara Sauce	1/2 Cup	70		Soy Sauce	1 Tbsp	8
Cocktail Sauce	2 Tbsp	30		Mayonnaise	1 Tbsp	90		Sriracha	1 Tbsp	5
Cranberry Sauce	2 Tbsp	50		Mustard	1 Tsp	3		Sugar	1 Tsp	16
Cinnamon	1 Tsp	6		Nutmeg	1 Tsp	12		Sweet and Sour Sauce	2 Tbsp	100
Eel Sauce	2 Tbsp	60		Onion Powder	1 Tsp	8		Sweet Chili Sauce	2 Tbsp	40
Garlic Powder	1 Tsp	10		Oregano	1 Tsp	5		Teriyaki Sauce	1 Tbsp	10
Garlic Salt	1 Tsp	5		Paprika	1 Tsp	6		Thousand Island Dressing	2 Tbsp	120
Ginger	1 Tbsp	18		Parsley	1 Tbsp	1		Tartar Sauce	2 Tbsp	140
Guacamole	2 Tbsp	45		Pepper	1 Tsp	5		Turmeric	1 Tsp	8
Honey	1 Tbsp	60		Pico de Gallo	2 Tbsp	10		Worcestershire Sauce	1 Tbsp	15
Honey Mustard	1 Tbsp	45		Ranch Dressing	2 Tbsp	140		Yum Yum Sauce	2 Tbsp	60

Fast Food

Ahhh, fast food. If you're like me, you love to eat out. If you're like me, cooking really isn't your thing. But you can still be successful on this diet even if you like to eat out. I have taken a couple of approaches.

1. I learned which fast foods wouldn't burn all of my calories for the day.
2. I saved fast foods for my cheat days on the weekends and tried to cook or buy convenient meals from the store during the week.

One thing to be careful of is the salads at big restaurant chains, as some of them have as many calories as a supersized Big Mac meal. This is particularly true if the salad contains breaded chicken. In this category especially, it bears repeating. Never eat anything without knowing its calorie content. Here are the charts for some common fast foods.

Burgers and Fries

(all burger calories are with cheese)

	Double Cheeseburger Name	Approx. Calories (Double)	Single Burger Name	Approx. Calories (Single)	Medium Fries	Approx. Calories
BURGER KING	Double Whopper	1040	Whopper	769	Fries	380
CARL'S JR. / HARDEE'S	Double Big Cheeseburger	760	Big Cheeseburger	540	Fries	420
CHECKERS / RALLY'S	Big Buford	660	Cheese Champ	430	Fries	500
CULVER'S	Culver's Deluxe Double	820	Culver's Deluxe Single	670	Fries	380
FIVE GUYS	Double Cheeseburger	980	Little Cheeseburger	610	Fries	953
IN-N-OUT BURGERS	Double-Double	610	Cheeseburger	430	Fries	395
KRYSTAL	Double Krystal with Cheese	300	Cheese Krystal	170	Fries	350
MCDONALD'S	Double Quarter Pounder	740	Quarter Pounder	520	Fries	378
MCDONALD'S	Double Cheeseburger	450	Cheeseburger	300	Fries	—
SHAKE SHACK	ShackBurger Double	760	ShackBurger	500	Fries	470
SONIC	SuperSonic Double Cheeseburger	1070	Sonic Cheeseburger	720	Fries	290
STEAK'N SHAKE	Double Steakburger with Cheese	640	Single Steakburger with Cheese	440	Fries	450
WAYBACK BURGERS	Classic Cheeseburger	650	Single Cheeseburger	350	Fries	520
WENDY'S	Dave's Double	888	Dave's Single	524	Fries	427
WHITE CASTLE	Double Cheese Slider	300	Cheese Slider	170	Fries	600

Chicken

	Chick-fil-A Calories	PDQ Calories	Zaxby's Calories	Church's Calories	KFC Calories	Popeyes Calories	McDonald's Calories	Wendy's Calories	Burger King Calories	Wingstop	Buffalo Wild Wings
Crispy Chicken Sandwich	420	490	780	650	650	700	470	490	600		
Grilled Chicken Sandwich	390	430	530	—	—	—	380	350	190		
Chicken Nuggets	250	340	—	160	300		250	222	224		
Chicken Tenders (3)	310	594	330	390	360	445					
Chicken Breast				250	390	380					
Chicken Leg				150	130	160					
Chicken Thigh				360	280	280					
Chicken Wing				290	130	210					
Sauced Wings or Tenders (1 order)		525	1000		1070	900		950		1300	720

Other Fast Food

RESTAURANT	FOOD	SERVING	CALORIES		RESTAURANT	FOOD	SERVING	CALORIES
Arby's	Classic Beef N Cheddar	1 sandwich	450		Nathan's Famous	Nathan's Deli Hotdog	1 hot dog	330
Arby's	Crispy Fish Sandwich	1 sandwich	570		Panda Express	Fried Rice	1 order	520
Burger King	Onion Rings	Medium	410		Panda Express	Orange Chicken	1 order	490
Burger King	Big Fish Sandwich	1 sandwich	570		Panda Express	Pot Stickers	3 potstickers	160
Charley's	Cheesesteak	Medium	750		Panda Express	Chinese Egg Roll	1 egg roll	200
Chick-Fil-A	Southwest Salad w/Dressing	1 order	630		Pizza Hut	Supreme Pizza	1 slice	305
Culver's	Cheese Curds	1 order	510		Popeyes	Classic Flounder Sandwich	1 sandwich	680
Culver's	North Atlantic Cod Filet Sandwich	1 sandwich	600		Portillo's	Chili Cheese Dog	1 hot dog	510
Domino's	Sausage Pizza	1 slice	311		Subway	Subway Club	6 inches	510
Hungry Howie's	Cheese Pizza	1 slice	200		Subway	Meatball Sub	6 inches	480
Japanese Restaurant	Shrimp Tempura Sushi	6 pieces	508		Taco Bell	Crunchy Taco Supreme	1 taco	190
McDonald's	Filet-O-Fish	1 sandwich	390		Taco Bell	Nachos BellGrande® – Beef	1 order	740
Moe's	Chicken Quesadilla	1 triangle	316		Taco Bell	Nacho Cheese – Plain	1 order	220

Strategies for Sticking to 1200 Calories

If you're going to start eating 1200 calories a day, you'll need to be strategic. Part of that is understanding exactly how you will stick to the diet. Here are some of my favorite strategies:

Keep Track of Favorite Low-Calorie Foods

As you eat 1200 calories day by day, you'll quickly learn your favorite low-calorie go-tos. My favorites included canned tuna (140 cals.), peanut butter and jelly sandwich (310), 10 pretzels filled with peanut butter (140), or a couple of boiled eggs (100). All of these are around 300 calories or less, immediately curb hunger, and help you easily make it to the next meal. Learn your favorites and make sure you always have those items on hand.

Intermittent Fasting

Intermittent fasting involves only eating within a certain time frame. A common fast includes the 16/8 method, which involves fasting for 16 hours and eating only during an 8-hour window. For example, you'd only eat between 10 a.m. and 6 p.m. or 12 p.m. and 8 p.m., etc. The time you choose is up to you. Just consider your schedule and identify the best time. Intermittent fasting automatically helps to restrict calories because you can only eat a certain number of calories within 8 hours.

One Meal a Day

This tactic is exactly as it sounds—eat just one meal a day. This is a great way to reduce calories because you can only eat so many calories in one sitting. The rest of the day, you can drink water, tea, or coffee. By the way, caffeine is also an excellent appetite suppressant. And don't be afraid to add a little honey if you need a little sweetener. One tablespoon is only 60 calories.

When I eat one meal a day, I also allow a small snack of around 200 or 300 calories. Now, the important thing about choosing this method is to know yourself. If eating one meal a day will cause you to consume 3000 calories when you finally do eat, it's not worth it. Also, experiment with what time to eat your one meal. If you choose to do it at breakfast, you'll likely find it hard to get through the rest of the day without eating much. Whenever I ate one meal a day, I had it no earlier than 4 p.m. Then I could have a light snack before bed if I got hungry.

Water Before Meals

If you are prone to overeating, one strategy is to drink a glass of water before each meal. Water is filling and will take up room in your stomach, automatically ensuring that you will eat fewer calories with each meal. Also remember, as stated earlier, water is just plain good for you overall, so getting more into your system is always a smart move.

Eat Constantly

This is the flip side of eating one meal a day. It involves eating multiple small meals throughout the day. It might seem counterintuitive to your goal, but hear me out. Many times if we deprive ourselves to the point where we're really hungry, we'll overeat at the next meal. That is why people who eat multiple meals often see success in their weight loss. They never get excessively hungry, so they never feel the need to overeat. Of course, you'll still need to keep calories in mind, which is why you need a list of low-calorie yet tasty options you can turn to when you need something to stave off hunger.

Save Most of Your Calories for the End of the Day

I found greater success when I ate lightly during the day and knew I could look forward to a meal of around 700 or

800 calories. Such a meal is largely satisfying, and consuming it near the end of the day will keep you feeling satisfied until bedtime, especially if you load up on protein and/or fiber. Think of it this way—if you have already consumed 800 calories by dinnertime, you only have 400 calories left to eat in the evening. That might be okay for you, but whenever I did this, I always wanted to eat a few more calories after dinner. So I'd end up consuming 1500 or 1600 calories for the day instead of 1200. It really just depends on how your brain works. My brain prefers to have dinner as my most satisfying meal. Your brain might be totally different, but you just need to experiment.

Load Up on Protein and Fiber

You don't want to start this diet and be hungry all the time. So protein and fiber will be your friend. Load up on these two every day and you'll find that a little food can go a long way. You'll feel full and be content until the next meal and won't have food on the brain all day. In addition to regular foods high in protein, there are countless other ways to get protein. There are protein chips, protein smoothies, shakes like Boost, and countless other protein snacks. Seriously, I think they have added protein to everything by now. A good brand to look for is Quest. And try to have protein at every meal, aiming at 70 to 80 grams for the day.

Purchase Prepackaged Meals

We touched on this earlier, but if you cook a lot at home, you may sometimes find that it's hard to judge the calories eaten. For example, say you cook a large pot of spaghetti sauce and noodles. Then you put some on a plate. You don't really have a good way of calculating the calories.

You could buy a food scale, but most people won't want the hassle. There's also the fact that cooking at home is just time-consuming, and many of us just don't have time to do it every day. Fortunately, there are alternatives.

Most grocery stores have a section near the meats or deli department with prepackaged dinners. And I'm not talking about frozen TV dinners (though you could get some of those too). You can get sides like mac & cheese or mashed potatoes and meat entrees like meatloaf or stuffed pork chops. You get the idea. The point is that these kinds of meals not only save you time but the calorie content is right on the package so you don't have to worry about figuring that out.

Chapter 5

Help! It's Not Working

So you began the 1200-calorie diet and a month or two later, you've lost little or no weight. First, know that this is highly unlikely, but it can happen. So what do you do? This diet should work for the average person, but there may be other factors at play if it doesn't. Following are some common reasons you just can't get rid of those pesky pounds.

You're Eating More Than 1200 Calories

Yeah, I know. This is soooooo obvious. But you'd be surprised how many people underestimate the calories they're eating. If you followed the instructions in this book, you should know exactly how many calories you're consuming each day. But mistakes happen. It's so easy to incorrectly calculate your calorie consumption. Maybe the calories listed for your favorite foods are only for one serving and you didn't realize there were actually four servings in the package. It's ok to eat more than one serving if that's what you decide. But you must always know exactly what you're eating and be sure to reflect that when logging your calories.

Another problem in calculating calories comes when you're eating something that's hard to calculate. We touched on this earlier. Maybe your mom makes her famous spaghetti once a week and you just can't resist it. And you can't accurately determine the calorie content without knowing all the ingredients and measurement amounts. However, you can use an app or the internet to get a good idea of calories per serving and at least be mindful of your portion size.

The same principle holds true when eating at restaurants. Don't overeat. Fortunately, restaurants are getting better at displaying the calories right on the menu, but you've still got to double-check. Are the calories listed for the entire meal or only a part of it? Always, always check serving sizes. Whenever I ate something I wasn't sure how to calculate, I just found the equivalent on MyFitnessPal or Google and used that number. Sometimes that's just the best you can do. But if you have to do this, err on the side of eating less rather than more.

You're Eating Less Than 1200 Calories

On the opposite end of the spectrum, you may be eating too little, which is causing your metabolism to slow down. I get it. Despite the warnings throughout this book, you thought you could speed things up a bit. After all, if eating 1200 calories is good for weight loss, then eating 800 must be even better. That sounds logical, and this will definitely work … initially. For a while. However, at some point, if you continue to significantly decrease your calorie intake, your body will try to conserve the little energy you give it.

That's why people starve themselves and still don't see the results they hope for. The body is trying to save itself! Unless you're under the care of a doctor who has a good reason for prescribing a lower-calorie diet, make sure you eat at least 1200 calories. It won't matter that much if you're short a day or two, but your body will think it has to fight to stay alive if you do this on a regular basis. Don't try to game the system. Eat a minimum of 1200 calories per day.

You're Impatient. It's Working ... Slowly

Do NOT read this book and expect the exact same results that I got. Your experience might mirror mine, but it's just as possible you will lose more or lose less. There are countless differences from person to person, and those differences influence the time it takes to lose weight. So don't chuck this book into the corner if you don't lose 40 pounds in 90 days. I've provided the details of my own journey as a guideline.

Judge your results by this one question: Are you losing weight month by month? Even if the scale doesn't show significant weight loss, are your clothes fitting better? If yes, then celebrate and be happy. The diet is working. There are more indicators of fitness than just numbers on a scale. You're doing fine. Keep on truckin'!

You're Gaining Muscle Faster Than You're Losing Fat

If you're exercising—especially if you're lifting weights— you're gaining muscle, which weighs more than fat. If you're gaining muscle faster than you're losing fat, it will appear that you're not losing weight. That's why some-times you must ignore the scale and pay more attention to what you see in the mirror. The scale might not reflect that you're losing fat and gaining muscle, but the mirror will! Your body will look more toned and your clothes will fit better. If you measure yourself, you may find that you have lost inches around your waist. If these things are happening but the scale isn't moving, don't worry. The scale will soon catch up to reality and begin to reflect the changes too.

You're Already at Optimal Weight

See, I knew it. You are one of THOSE people. Just stubborn! At the beginning of this book, didn't I tell you to keep it moving if you're already a perfect 10 and trying to lose two pounds of belly fat? And now here you are, wondering why you're not losing weight. You might *want* to lose weight, but that doesn't necessarily mean you *need* to. The 1200-cal-orie diet works best for those who are significantly over-weight. If you already weigh what you should and you begin a 1200-calorie diet, your body will likely go into en-ergy conservation mode, preventing you from losing weight.

Or maybe that's not your situation. You were obedient! You followed the steps in this book correctly and lost some weight. But maybe the goal weight you initially set is too low for your body type. Remember that online weight cal-culators are only estimates and can't possibly take into ac-count all the unique properties of your body. Suppose the calculations indicated you should weigh 150, but you get to 160 and can't lose any more. You've tried everything and nothing works. But despite not being able to reach your goal weight, you look great. In that case, maybe 160 is your optimal weight rather than 150. Always be willing to adjust if you need to. You might even get to 170 and conclude that you like the way you look. That's ok too. You can decide when to stop. It's your body. You decide what looks good on you. Don't let the scale rule your life.

You're Retaining Water

Sometimes you can eat the correct number of calories, but your diet consists of things that cause you to retain water, namely excess carbs and sodium. Evaluate your calorie log for the past week and see whether you've been exceeding the recommended intake for carbs or sodium. If so, cut back and see if there's a change. Additionally, it may seem coun-terintuitive to drink more water if you're retaining it, but drinking more does help. If you don't drink enough water, your body might decide to hold on to what's already in your system. If you think this might be the problem, see if increasing your water intake helps.

You've Hit a Weight-Loss Plateau

It happens to all of us. You've been losing weight quite nicely, thank you very much, and then suddenly, nothing. Week after week, you step onto the scale and there's no pro-gress, even though the effort level is the same. Is the scale broken? Probably not. You've just hit the dreaded weight loss plateau. A weight-loss plateau can occur even when you're doing all the things you were doing before.

There are two main solutions to the problem of the weight loss plateau. And the first one is fun:

1. **Eat!** That's right. Take two days and eat what you want. Don't count any calories. Let your body know that you're not really trying to starve it. Most of the time that will be enough to break through the plateau and get your metabolism going again. If it's not, try a longer duration, like a week.

2. **Exercise.** If you're not already exercising, start doing so. If you're already exercising, change it up a bit. Your body can get used to a particular workout routine and cease burning calories as effectively as it used to. Try some different exercises and/or different or more strenuous exercise routines. Adding exercise to the equation revs up your metabolism so you can begin losing weight again. And remember, walking *does* count as exercise.

3. **Add Weights**. If you're already eating the right number of calories and exercising, then try adding weights. Weight training helps you burn calories even when you're not exercising. So you'll start burning more calories while doing things like watching TV or sleeping, and who wouldn't love that?

Each time you hit a plateau, employ one of these remedies as many times as necessary until you've met your goal weight. I believe I avoided reaching a plateau precisely because I purposely took breaks from the plan. When I came back, my body was ready to resume weight loss because it knew I wasn't trying to starve it.

If you're in the middle of a weight-loss plateau, don't stress too much about it. Weight loss is a process. You may lose nothing for three weeks and then suddenly lose four pounds in one week. Plateaus are discouraging and stressful, but don't let it get to you. Just keep remembering that the scale is only one indicator of physical fitness.

You're Weighing Yourself Too Often

Earlier, I suggested weighing yourself once a week rather than once a day, but some of you got too excited and weighed yourself once a day anyway. Trust me, I understand the compulsion. But doing this can also make it appear that your weight loss has slowed wayyyyy down—even if it hasn't. Remember, it can take a whole week to lose one or two pounds, so of course, some days you will get on the scale and see the same number over and over again. That's because you've lost a quarter of a pound or something like that, which won't really show up on a scale. And if you're weighing yourself once a week and the numbers start making you too crazy, weigh in once a month instead.

Your Metabolism Is Slow for Medical Reasons

If you've made multiple adjustments and the 1200-calorie diet still isn't working, it's time for a trip to the doctor's office. Get a physical and find out if there's a reason your metabolism is slow. Common reasons for slow weight loss include a thyroid condition or menopause, but there are many other medical causes as well. Only a doctor can tell you for sure.

Chapter 6

What's Exercise Got to Do With It?

I know, I know. You feel tricked, deceived! The title of this book said NOTHING about exercise, and now here's a chapter on it. Well, hold on a sec and allow me to ease your mind right up front. You *do not* have to exercise for the 1200-calorie diet to work. Not at all. You *can* still lose weight without it. I promise. I've done it.

The reason you don't have to exercise for this to work is simple. When people exercise for weight loss, they do it to ensure they're burning more calories than they're consuming. But when you're on a 1200-calorie diet, you're already eating at a deficit simply by going about your daily activities. Put another way, people on this diet are already burning far more calories than they consume, so exercise is just a bonus.

Here's a quick recap to ease your mind. Remember earlier you calculated your BMR and that told you how many calories your body needs to sustain itself. For most people, that number fell somewhere between 1800 and 2500. But now you're eating 1200 calories. That means you're already operating at a deficit of, at minimum, 600 calories a day. That's why exercise isn't necessary for you to lose weight.

So if you don't want to exercise, you may now do the happy dance and skip this chapter. But you've already made it this far, so you might as well stay with me. The chapter is fairly short, and you might change your mind.

Why Exercise?

Exercising isn't necessary to lose weight, but that doesn't mean it's not beneficial in a myriad of other ways. And I know I'm telling you something you already know. You've heard all your life that exercise is important! Losing weight is definitely a benefit, but exercise also provides energy, dulls hunger, increases metabolism, keeps the heart healthy, fights off depression, and builds muscle.

If your goal is weight loss only, do the 1200-calorie diet and laugh diabolically as you pass by the folks slaving away in the gym. But if your goal is to be healthy, actually change your body shape, or get toned, you'll have to incorporate exercise. Yeah. Sorry. A calorie deficit will make you lose weight, but only exercise can sculpt your body into a more pleasing shape. You can weigh 180 and be flabby or you can weigh 180 and be toned. And there's a huge visible difference between the two.

Adding exercise was a no-brainer for me. It made me feel good physically and mentally, and I knew I wanted both weight loss and body sculpting. I wanted results fast, and I wanted to do everything I could to increase my chances of success. So a few months into my journey on the 1200-calorie diet, I worked with a personal trainer two days a week for strength training—yep, that included weights! I also exercised on my own for the rest of the week, primarily with aerobic videos.

Adding exercise to your weight loss strategy improves your odds of getting the results you want, and I highly recommend it. You don't even have to start exercising right away. You can add it at any point in your plan. And you don't need a personal trainer. Initially, just start walking every day and then escalate from there. Exercise videos provide workouts at various levels and durations. Don't laugh, but I'm partial to Richard Simmons' (RIP) *Sweatin' to the Oldies* videos. They're just plain fun and they make me feel like I'm dancing, not working out! It's a four-set series, and all but the first one are available on YouTube.

There are also many trainers on YouTube who provide short, equipment-free workouts that you can do at home. Try channels like MadFit or PS Fit if you're looking for a traditional workout or The Fitness Marshall if you want to do some dancing. Eventually, you can add weight or resistance training for even better results.

Start where you can and build from there. A good guideline is to start at 15 minutes a day and increase to at least 30 or 45 minutes, which is the length of an average exercise session. Also, exercise can be done in chunks throughout the day. Maybe you dread the idea of spending 45 minutes exercising, but you don't mind fitting in two 20-minute sessions.

Even if you don't want to start an official exercise plan, you can do the following to begin incorporating more activity into your life and accelerating your weight loss results:

- Park a considerable distance away from the entrance when going to work or to the store.

- Get up often to walk around and stretch during the day.
- Choose the restroom furthest away from your desk.
- Participate in bowling or other sports you enjoy at least once a week.
- Take the stairs rather than the elevator.
- Download an app that tracks your steps and make a game of beating yourself each week.
- Take a short walk after every meal.

You can add more activity to your lifestyle gradually until you are ready to begin an exercise plan. Also note that a group activity may motivate you more, so check around for exercise classes offered at the YMCA, your gym, or via private trainers. Some are even free.

The Benefits of Weight Training

Building muscle is the absolute best way to change the way your body looks, and the best way to build muscle is via strength training. Yep, you've got to pick up some weights, but they don't have to be very heavy. Such training develops strength in the body's core muscle groups. It involves lifting, pushing, or pulling weights in a series of repetitions at various and often increasing weight loads. Strength training can be accomplished using your own body weight (think push-ups or sit-ups) or by using dumbbells or weightlifting machines.

The benefits include improvement in flexibility, metabolic rate, bone density, physical strength, muscle tone, and overall appearance. The more muscle you develop, the more fat you burn, even when you're not exercising. And who doesn't want that kind of benefit? Weight training also helps prevent the loss of muscle tissue that commonly occurs with age. When you lose weight, you can lose both fat and muscle. Weight training is the best way to ensure that you lose the fat and keep the muscle. Here's the bottom line. Do you want some curves where there are none? Gotta strength train.

Keep Track of Calories Burned

If you decide to exercise, keep track of the calories burned so you can log that information in your fitness app. On the 1200-calorie diet, you're already keeping track of *calories in*. In this step, you're going to keep track of *calories out*. You don't *have* to do this, because being on the 1200-calorie diet really is enough. However, there are some benefits to keeping track of this data. The main reason is that it always helps to have all the data possible available to you. There are a few ways you can calculate calories burned:

- **Estimate it**. You can look up various workouts in your app or on the internet. When you select an activity, the program will give you a projected number of calories burned. But when you use this method, the calorie expenditure is only an estimate and will likely be off by a significant degree.

- **Rely on gym equipment**. Most gym equipment like an exercise bike, elliptical machine, or treadmill will keep track of your calorie expenditure for you. Some machines will have you input your weight and age; others just require you to periodically grab the handles to read your heart rate. This method is more accurate than the first, but it's still not exact. In my experience, the machines overstate the calories burned by about 100. Plus, when you switch to weight training, you'll have to go back to estimating, as the weight training machines don't calculate calories burned.

- **Wear a heart rate monitor, FitBit, or other Smart Watch during exercise**. This is my preference because it's the best way to get a true reading of the calories burned—whether you're at home or at the gym, whether you're doing aerobic or weight training activity. A good monitor will run you about $70 to $200, but it's worth the money. Estimating calorie expenditure in one of the two ways above is adequate when you first get started, but you will eventually require a more accurate reading, especially as your weight loss begins to slow down. Monitoring your exercise calorie expenditure is always a good place to start if diet alone stops producing results.

Logging calories burned is important to your success. If you don't know how many calories you're currently burning, you won't be able to adjust if the need arises. You need that information in order to accurately monitor your progress.

Should You Replace the Calories Burned?

So you started the 1200-calorie diet and decided to add exercise to your weight loss plan. Let's say you eat 1200 calories and burn 500 calories through exercise. For the day, this gives you a net calorie balance of 700 calories. Should you eat another 500 calories to replace what you burned and get the total back up to 1200? My overall answer is no because that will give you the fastest benefits. However, my other answer is it really depends on your body and what you can tolerate. There's no right or wrong answer. You will lose weight whether you eat the extra 500 calories or not, but one way is definitely faster than the other. Here are some questions to ask to help you make the decision:

1. **Am I too weak after or during exercise?** If you are, go ahead and eat all or some of the calories you burned to replenish your strength.

2. **Am I too hungry after exercise?** If you are, go ahead and eat. Remember, you don't want to feel you're depriving yourself. You don't want hunger pains to drive you to binge eating. But try a snack first, not a full-course meal. You may be surprised at how little you need.

3. **Do I want to eat the extra calories just because I can?** If that's the case, you have my blessing. Eat up! Some people exercise just so they can eat! And I ain't mad at 'em. I've done the same.

However, if there are no adverse effects and you can handle it, I recommend not replacing the calories burned. To be clear. If you eat 1200 calories and burn 500, I think you should leave it at that. Remember, *when* you eat doesn't matter, so you can definitely plan your meals so that you can eat after your workout. You might plan breakfast after your morning workout or your dinner or a snack after your evening workout.

MyFitnessPal used to encourage me to eat whatever extra calories I burned. I told my trainer and he said, "No, absolutely not." So I did it his way and was pleased with the results. It may or may not work for you. Most days, I burned 400 to 500 calories through exercise and close to 800 on weight training days. For the most part, I didn't replace the calories I burned. And that definitely helped me lose more than if I had eaten the extra calories. I still had a lot of energy, I felt good, and I wasn't hungry. In many cases, exercising actually suppressed my appetite. But if I wanted to eat something extra, I had some leeway to do so. And sometimes I did, but even then, I would only eat an extra 200 calories or so.

But everyone is different. I was never really hungry on the 1200-calorie diet. In fact, I initially had trouble getting to 1200! My daughter often makes fun of me because she says I can get full just by eating a grape. And that's only a slight exaggeration. I don't require a lot of food to feel satisfied. My problem has never been the need to eat a lot of food; my problem is that I like to eat out and I like foods that are high in calories.

Just know that if you decide to replace the calories you burn, you're not cheating. Eat 'em if you want, and don't feel guilty. You're still on the 1200-calorie diet; you're just accomplishing it by eating 1700 calories and burning off the extra 500 calories. Do what works for you. Do whatever will make life easier while staying within the guidelines and your diet will be a success. Not replacing those calories burned worked well for me, and my pounds melted away! But do what feels best to you! [*Just don't eat 1700 calories knowing full well you aren't burning off 500 (-; *].

Chapter 7

To 1200 Calories and Beyond! Increasing Calories Without Gaining Weight

Y ou did it! You started the 1200-calorie diet and watched the weight fall off as if by magic. Well, allow me to give you a huge congratulations! You've worked so hard to get to this point, and you should be very proud of yourself. This journey isn't an easy one, and the fact that you didn't give up is a testament to your strength.

But here's the thing. 1200 calories a day isn't meant to be a permanent lifestyle change. It's meant to kickstart your weight loss efforts. So that means the journey's not over once you've lost the weight. Now you've got to learn how to keep it off while increasing your caloric intake. So let's walk through how to adjust to a normal routine after following the 1200-calorie diet.

Beginning to Eat Normally Again

I know exactly what you're thinking. Once you've reached your goal weight and begin eating normally again, won't you start gaining weight? It's a reasonable assumption, but no, you really shouldn't gain any if you begin eating at your calorie **maintenance level**. That's the key. You can't start overeating; you've got to eat to maintain and not to gain. Remember, your maintenance level is the number of calories you burn just by existing day by day.

On the 1200-calorie diet, you were operating at a significant calorie deficit. You were giving your body *less* energy than it needed to function. This deficit was causing your weight loss. Now you need to give your body *exactly* the amount of energy it needs to function. Remember the rule: Consume more calories than you burn and you'll gain weight. Burn more calories than you consume and you'll lose weight. And if your calorie expenditure and calorie consumption balance out, you'll maintain your weight.

So once you reach your ideal weight, you should be able to easily return to the normal caloric intake for your height and body weight. You'll simply stop losing and begin maintaining your current weight. Remember, I took several breaks while on the 1200-calorie diet, but during those breaks, I still maintained my weight. That's because even though I was eating more, I wasn't eating so much that my caloric consumption was higher than my caloric output.

As you increase your calories, it's important to keep logging them, both in and out. This may seem annoying, but you don't want to risk undoing all of your hard work. It's easier than you might think to slip back into the habit of mindless snacking or repeatedly ordering delicious, calorie-dense meals from your favorite restaurant. You owe it to yourself to make sure the results you worked for don't disappear. Remember the benefits of mindful eating! You need to continue cultivating a good relationship with food if you want to keep the weight off and feel your best.

Keep in mind that when you reach your ideal weight, you'll need to recalculate your BMR and BMI to determine your new maintenance level. And if you're worried about increasing your calorie intake, you can do so gradually until you reach maintenance. Be as mindful of this process as you were when you first began your diet. As you know, the calories—and your weight— can creep up before you know it.

Don't Be Discouraged

Don't lose hope if your results aren't what you expect. Unless you're using a fitness app that records both your calorie intake and expenditure, you can only get an estimate of your maintenance level. The best indicator of what you should or should not do is your body's response. Don't be afraid to make adjustments if necessary. If you calculate your BMR and your new maintenance level is 1900, eat at that level for several weeks and evaluate. Are you losing weight? Then increase your daily calorie intake by 200 for a few weeks. Are you gaining weight? Then decrease by 200 calories and see how that works. Are you maintaining your weight? Great! That means you've found your magic calorie number. Continually evaluate your progress and note any weight fluctuations. You worked hard to lose the weight, so don't let it creep up on you again.

Keep Working Toward Your Goals

Now is a good time to revisit your long-term goals. Are you taking a break before starting the whole weight loss process over again, or are you satisfied with what you accomplished? Whatever the case, be proud of yourself. Celebrate your progress and continue to work toward your goals.

Chapter 8

That's All, Folks!

Remember that 1200 calories is only a guideline. It's not meant to make you a slave to a caloric intake that doesn't work for you. For various reasons, you may require a different number, and that's ok. You must evaluate your present condition, set goals based on where you want to be, and then determine the best way to get there. Don't give up if this exact plan doesn't work for you. Keep adapting until you find something that *does* work.

I hope you learned a lot from this book and that it will help you lose weight and keep it off. More than that, though, I hope you'll work to set yourself up for success in other ways as well. Remember the importance of your mental and emotional well-being when it comes to reducing cravings and increasing your overall life satisfaction. If you were feeling overwhelmed before picking up this book, I hope I've been able to grant you some peace along your weight loss journey. Overall, I hope you feel energized and determined now that you're armed with the knowledge to help you improve your health.

Now you have a choice. You can decide that I'm some crazy chick and ignore the advice in this book. Or you can try it for a month and see if it works. You can start slowly, decreasing your calorie intake little by little until you get down to 1200 calories. It's all up to you. Maybe you're skeptical that it will work. But what if it does? Then you will have succeeded where you've often failed before. So give it a chance. You've got absolutely nothing to lose … except those pesky pounds.

Happy dieting! :)

List of Links

ere's a handy list of all the websites mentioned in this book.

NOTE: If you're reading the print book, please visit https://1200caloriediet.net/book-links **for easy access to all the links below.**

Website Links

1200CalorieDiet.Net
Facebook.com/The1200CalorieDiet
https://1200caloriediet.net/book-links
https://1200caloriediet.net/downloads/

Fitness Calculators and Recording

BMI Calculator
BMR Calculator
https://www.myfitnesspal.com/

Food Delivery Services

https://www.homechef.com/
https://www.factor75.com/

1200-Calorie Meal Plans
- Good Housekeeping: A 7-Day, 1,200-Calorie Weight Loss Meal Plan
- National Heart Lung and Blood Institute: Traditional American Cuisine: 1,200 Calories
- Eating Well: Simple 1200-Calorie Meal Plan

YouTube Fitness Videos
MadFit
PS Fit
The Fitness Marshall

Enjoyed the book?
Please leave a review on your favorite book-buying platform.

www.ingramcontent.com/pod-product-compliance
Lightning Source LLC
Chambersburg PA
CBHW060511280326
41933CB00014B/2925